# TOOLS
# FOR
# PRIMARY
# CARE
# RESEARCH

*EDITED BY*

*MOIRA STEWART*
*FRED TUDIVER*
*MARTIN J. BASS*
*EARL V. DUNN*
*PETER G. NORTON*

**Research Methods**
**for Primary Care**
*Volume 2*

**SAGE** Publications
*International Educational and Professional Publisher*
Newbury Park   London   New Delhi

*For information address*:

 SAGE Publications, Inc.
2455 Teller Road
Newbury Park, California 91320

SAGE Publications Ltd.
6 Bonhill Street
London EC2A 4PU
United Kingdom

SAGE Publications India Pvt. Ltd.
M-32 Market
Greater Kailash I
New Delhi 110 048 India

Printed in the United States of America

**Library of Congress Cataloging-in-Publication Data**

Main entry under title:

Tools for primary care research/ edited by Moira A. Stewart. . . [et al.].
        p.   cm.   —(Research methods for primary care ; v. 2)
    Includes bibliographical references and index.
    ISBN 0-8039-4403-9.   — ISBN 0-8039-4404-7 (pbk.)
    1. Medicine—Research—Methodology.   I. Stewart, Moira.
II. Series.
RA440.T59    1992
610'.72—dc20                                           92-2706

92   93   94   95   1   2   3   4   5   6   7   8   9   10   11

Sage Production Editor: Diane S. Foster

# Contents

# Foreword

## JOHN HOWIE

This book is the second of six on the foundations of primary care research. Its 20 chapters capture something of the breadth and depth of expertise of primary care research and reflect the largely expanding professionalism in this growing area of sociomedical endeavor. This foreword attempts to give flesh to the bones of the book and to reflect its hidden, as well as its formal, agenda that together will make reading it an enjoyable and rewarding experience.

## The Formal Agenda

The formal agenda of the book offers the two key introduction chapters, a series of chapters on basic concepts, basic techniques, tools for measurement, data collection, and data analysis. The authors are researchers of high repute.

## Context: A Basic Research Tool

This book makes an assumption that the reader shares basic research competences and experiences: "Intellectual organization." This was in fact the theme of the first book of this series and is such a key "tool" in the building of rewarding and effective research that it is necessary to restate some of the basic ground rules somewhere within this book so that readers visiting this text in isolation from the others in the series can recognize the common ground from which all critical inquiry starts and on which all research is thus built.

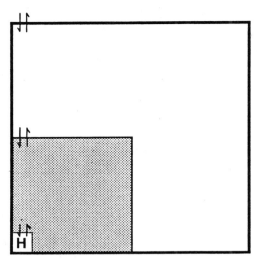

**Figure 1.** Episode of Illness Cared for in the Hospital (H), General Practice
          (shaded area), and Outside Formal Professional Services (white area)

Where are we starting from? What have we already available? Why are
we where we are? What do we need to move forward? Figure 1 shows the
well-known simple portrayal of the relationship between the pathology-
rich area of hospital medicine, the more unstructured bio-psycho-social
domain of general practice or family medicine, and the still less defined
outer area, which contains three quarters of health problems that are
really variants of the state of health or the state of illness. Outside the
figure lies the field of wellness, probably unattainable in terms of the
World Health Organization's credo of "complete mental, physical and
social well-being," but real for many and the target of all who work in
the medical and social sciences.

Four principal actors determine where and why the play takes place.
In the simplest terms (Figure 2) the actors are "the illness," "the patient,"
"the doctor" (or other formal or informal caretakers), and "the family."
Each of these can be expanded almost endlessly, as the illness is divided
by its pathologies (biomedical or psychosocial) or its symptoms; the
patient and the doctor are defined in terms of their cultures (for example,
their health beliefs, expectations, wants, and needs); and the family is
seen first in terms of its conventional nuclear and biologically linked
members and then in the wider context of community.

When these are interlinked as in Figure 2, family or community is
given centrality, and so judgments are made of the relative importance

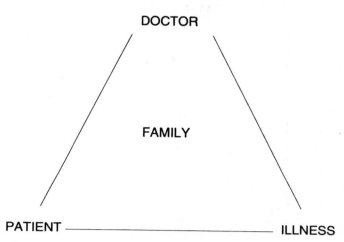

**Figure 2.** Issues in a Patient's Health

of any of the other major issues that will be working at one time (or at one consultation or in any interaction).

Figures 1 and 2 form one vision of the key elements of the "grounded theory" that is often referred to: They have the merits of simplicity (but not triviality) at one end, and of infinite variety and complexity at the other. They provide a map or framework for those setting out on the journey— or temporarily lost en route.

Once "context" has been defined, many researchers (although not all) would agree that two steps are needed: A question has to be asked, and a search for a numerator and a denominator begun. The question should interest and feel important to the researcher, and—reflecting at least my own vision of what research is about and for—attempt to promote understanding of or solutions to issues or problems that are personal to the researcher. This step, if properly done, substantially lessens the risk of undertaking the collection of irrelevant information, which so devalues the research process when it happens. And the research question should preferably be either an answerable one or one capable of being divided step by step into portions that can be wrestled with in turn.

## The Hidden Agenda

All books have a second or hidden agenda, and this one is no exception. The tension between quantitative and qualitative research (not so

much as methodologies but more in terms of the researchers themselves), which had become the polarizing feature of the first book of the
series, simmers near the surface for this book. At times this tension is or
has been creative, but it seems desirable to resolve it before it detracts
from the common ground of both approaches and impedes the processes
of the three next books in the series.

The first step toward resolution is to recognize that the stereotypes of
the two modes do not hold up. The quantitative camp is no more the
domain of reductionists and doctors and those who engage in "count-
ing," than is the qualitative camp the habitat of social scientists and
those who engage in "thinking." The reality is that the large majority of
those who research effectively in primary care want to create change and
want to base the campaign for change on arguments that have real
understanding and meaning to underpin them. Feinstein's writings (1972)
were quoted in support of both starting positions. Is his plea for basing
progress on "the judgments of thoughtful people" the way ahead? A
judgment requires balancing choices, and balancing means weighing
not always on an ordinal scale but often in a categorical mode. It is the
word *thoughtful* that can do most to help. The uniting theme is rejection
of the authoritarian and simplistic teachings and practice of what is, it
is to be hoped, a past school of medical educators and politicians in the
reductionist mode. The need is to recognize that all effective research
will have phases of both qualitative development and the use of quantitative skills interwoven throughout its planning, its carrying out, and
its analysis, interpretation, and dissemination.

If step one has been to recognize that "quantitative" and "qualitative"
are not on parallel nonconverging tramlines, step two seems to be to
move from placing these approaches as polar points on a line to putting
them in a continuous feedback loop one with another (Figure 3). Then
the tools that this book describes can be seen to be the common property
they surely are. The challenge is for researchers to drop their stereotyp-
ing of each other, to enter the circle, and to use these tools constructively
and in partnership.

The tools this book is concerned with are evolving fast to meet the
needs of those doing research in primary care. The book has attempted
to give some structure to the issues it considers by devoting sections to
concepts and issues, to basic techniques, to tools that can be used to collect
information, and to tools that can be used to measure the issues of importance in our field. Some chapters could equally be placed in a different
section, and several necessarily discuss issues (particularly reliability
and validity) already developed by different contributors. Thus both the

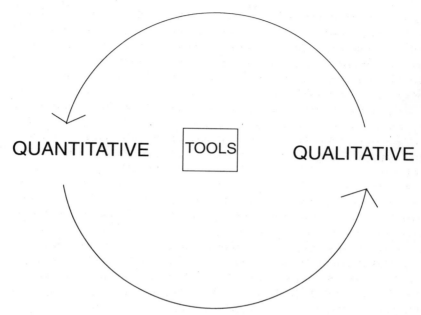

**Figure 3.** The Relationship between Qualitative and Quantitative Research

individuality and the continuity of ideas, authors, and researchers are given their place.

## Overview

Hames and Metcalfe offer the key chapters. The first is a poetic journey through three decades of the work of a solo family physician with a feel for the importance of observation and the questioning of the unexpected. This is a story of the place of individualism and of its enhancement by wise use of the expertise of others and collaboration with them. The second is a thoughtful, scholarly, and visionary exposition of the challenges facing primary care research as it attempts to define desired outcomes of care and to improve care by measuring these outcomes and responding to what we find. It is academic in the best sense of the word.

Many who read or dip in and out of this text will have read John Berger's (1976) story of a country doctor, *A Fortunate Man*. Its opening lines are infinitely requotable: "Landscapes can be deceptive. Sometimes a landscape seems to be less a setting for the life of its inhabitants than a curtain

behind which their struggles, achievements and accidents take place"
(Berger, 1976, inside cover).

At one level this book is about landscapes, about recognizing that they
change with the season and with the weather and are seen differently
by different people, and about recognizing the role of different ways of
portraying these landscapes, such as by word, paint, or photograph. At
a second level the story is about the extra rewards of seeing behind the
curtain and recognizing that those who look can see only what they can
understand, that understanding comes from having insights and skills
that also feed from each other.

## References

Berger, J. M. H. (1976). *A fortunate man*. London: Writers & Readers.
Feinstein, A. R. (1972). The need for humanised science in evaluating medication. *Lancet*,
    2, 421.

# Acknowledgments

This book and the series owe a debt to the Physicians Services Incorporated Foundation, which saw a need to strengthen the resources for researchers in primary care and chose to fund this project.

This book would not have come about without the commitment of two groups: The Centre for Studies in Family Medicine of The University of Western Ontario, London, Ontario; and the Primary Care Research Unit of Sunnybrook Health Science Centre, North York, Ontario. Drs. Brian Hennen and Ian McWhinney have inspired Drs. Stewart and Bass in their initiatives on behalf of primary care research. Drs. Tudiver, Dunn, and Norton want to thank Sunnybrook, their hospital, and especially the physicians in the Department of Family and Community Medicine for their continued support, understanding, and patience.

While this book was in preparation, Dr. Stewart was a Career Scientist of the Ontario Ministry of Health, Health Research Personnel Development Program.

We are indebted to Anne Stilman for her excellent editing of the manuscript.

We thank Jane Wood for coordinating this project and typing the manuscripts.

"The Island of Research Map" by Ernest Harbury is reproduced by permission of *American Scientist* and the author.

# Series Editors' Introduction

This book is Volume 2 in the series Foundations of Primary Care Research. It provides a counterbalance to the more conceptual Volume 1. A number of chapters on principles and guidelines are presented for the more thoughtful investigator, but it is mainly a "how to" guide related to primary care research. After reading Volume 1 on traditional and innovative approaches, the researcher will be well prepared to select both the approach and the design that are appropriate to the well-honed research question. The researcher then confronts the realities of how to proceed with data collection and analysis. Volume 2, *Tools for Primary Care Research*, addresses many important issues at this stage of the research process.

Moira Stewart
Peter G. Norton
Fred Tudiver
Martin J. Bass
Earl V. Dunn

# Introduction

MOIRA STEWART

In our thinking about the role of research in the disciplines of primary care, we have been challenged by the writings of Ravetz (1971) regarding disciplines that are on the road to maturity. Our discipline will become mature only when a "mass of positive knowledge" exists. This book encourages such a development. The kinds of knowledge that are not yet available to primary care practitioners and that it is incumbent on us researchers to provide include incidence and prevalence of conditions and presenting complaints, the patients' experiences of the illness, relationships with the family, the natural history of common problems, the accuracy of diagnostic tests in the primary care setting, the patients' ideas and beliefs about health problems and therapy, the health care system, and the effect of interventions for conditions of interest to primary care practitioners.

How can primary care research become as strong as necessary to help lead the discipline to maturity? What are the components of the research process that must be addressed? One could argue that many exist, but two in particular are met by this book.

The first component—the tools of research—is explicitly addressed and is the central topic of this book. While the foundation of a project is the research question and the blueprint is the design chosen to answer that question, the tools are the bricks, mortar, hammers, and lathes. Without these, even the most elegantly designed structures do not rise above the foundations. In addition, because tools come in many sizes, shapes, and colors, they must be selected with care or the edifice will be cockeyed.

The second component of the research process, implicitly addressed by this book, concerns the education of primary care researchers. The intent is to discuss models of excellent primary care research by including chapters written by internationally renowned primary care scholars who have vast experience and who share their projects and interests with us. We can be encouraged and guided by their example. Our discipline will become mature only when we cease to be distracted by controversies about worthy fundamental approaches, valid research problems, and acceptable methods. This book provides examples of different approaches addressing a variety of relevant primary care problems using a plethora of methods. Our purpose in presenting qualitative and quantitative tools side by side is to stress that, as primary care researchers, we should take off the blinders. We must open our minds to all available approaches and methods in order to select those best suited to our current research topic. Maturity will require the development of the tools and techniques to enable the investigator to get on with the job. This book directly sets out to provide the reader with some of these tools.

The first two chapters are inspirational offerings from two world-famous primary care researchers: Curtis G. Hames, from the United States; and David Metcalfe, from Great Britain.

Chapters 3 to 6 comprise Part I. In Chapter 3 a Canadian family practice researcher, Martin J. Bass, makes the case that the most basic tools in primary care research are the clinician-researchers themselves. On their self-knowledge and observational abilities all else rests. In the next chapter Maurice Wood, a founding father of United States family medicine research, provides a next step for the clinician-researcher, a method for classifying clinical encounters that has been tested in primary care settings around the world. Next, David Wilkin, noted British sociologist, presents the reader with principles for selecting measures of outcomes in clinical practice. Finally, Lorraine E. Ferris and Peter G. Norton elucidate two particular principles for assessing measures: reliability and validity.

Part II of the book contains three important "how to" chapters. Truls Østbye, a Norwegian epidemiologist now in Canada, outlines the decisions that are required when a researcher selects a sample of patients. Fred Tudiver and Lorraine E. Ferris provide a step-by-step guide to creating a new measure. This chapter is best read in conjunction with Chapters 5 and 6. In Chapter 9 Stephen J. Zyzanski gives another side of the picture provided by Tudiver and Ferris. He suggests appropriate techniques and standards for making new measures from old ones. Zyzanski presents some very pertinent data on the effect of the number of items in a measure on its reliability and the effects of reliability on validity.

The nine chapters in Parts III, IV, and V describe tools of measurement, data collection, and data analysis. Larry Culpepper, a past president of the North American Primary Care Research Group (NAPCRG), focusing on pain, writes about measures of symptoms that are relevant to primary care studies. A review of quality-of-life measures is presented by Canadian sociologist J. Ivan Williams, while in Chapter 12 Cindy I. Carlson provides an overview of measures to assess families. A well-tested and widely used measure of functional status, called the COOP chart, is given in Chapter 13 by an American primary care research team including David W. Beaufait, a family practitioner from New Hampshire.

Space limitations allowed us to present only three tools for data collection. First the scholars Richard A. MacLachlan and Brian Hennen write about the medical record as the source of data and the audit as a tool to abstract the data. Second, in Chapter 15, David L. Morgan reviews the central issues in conducting a study employing focus groups. He provides a number of examples of such work that are relevant to practitioners in primary care. Third, William L. Miller and Benjamin F. Crabtree, United States proponents of qualitative methods in primary care research, give guidelines for engaging in long open-ended interviews.

Two tools for data analysis are included in Chapters 17 and 18. Crabtree and Miller demystify the analysis of transcripts of text from long interviews in the first of these chapters. Subsequently Peter G. Norton, Edmee Franssen, and Earl V. Dunn give a thoughtful guide to helping select computer software for analyzing data.

Finally, and perhaps one of the most valuable parts of this book, is the Inventory of Psychosocial Measurement Instruments Useful in Primary Care, found in the Appendix. Scott H. Frank, along with members of the Society of Teachers of Family Medicine, compiled this annotated bibliography of instruments to measure many constructs relevant to primary care, including social support, alcoholism, marital satisfaction, anxiety, and health-risk behavior.

The purpose of this book is not so much to help contemplate research as it is to aid in *doing* research. We hope that this book will assist readers in the conduct and completion of their research projects.

## References

Ravetz, J. R. (1971). *Scientific knowledge and its social problems.* New York: Oxford University Press.

# 1 In the Eyes of the Beholder: A Thirty-Year Odyssey of Research in Primary Care

CURTIS G. HAMES

## Introduction

It is a privilege to have this opportunity to share some of the thoughts and exciting experiences that, as a country doctor, I have derived from research in family medicine. My goal here is not to discuss methodology, which is covered in other chapters, but to expand the horizon of the opportunities for research that are becoming more apparent almost daily in your own practices. To recognize and appreciate these new opportunities, we must understand where they are coming from and how they relate to the whole. Since this chapter represents only one dimension in an anticipated series of volumes devoted to the many parameters of research in primary care, it would appear appropriate, first, to place it in its proper context.

My discussions with students and faculty members in many parts of the world have suggested a lack of clear understanding in several areas concerning the nature of research in primary care. The first area for further classification concerns the need to appreciate the important resources and potential contribution that every practitioner has at his or her command. In particular, opportunities exist for participation at different levels of involvement in the research process. Each component of a research project is equally important to the success of the whole. Often we have access to certain populations or diseases that are denied to the bench scientist who in turn has special talents or equipment we do not have. Yet even today, in large university medical centers, I see many research projects suffering for the want of such cooperation. Do not hesitate, if possible, to provide the missing link to make a research project possible.

After 30 years of practical experience, I have developed what I call the anatomy of a research project, which I hope will help encourage such cooperation. A primary care clinician can engage in four levels of commitment, as follows:

*Level 1* represents a complete commitment: providing the original idea, conducting a review of the literature, developing the hypothesis and research plans, selecting the instruments of assessment, securing funding, personally managing the data collection and analysis, preparing the write-up, and securing its publication.*The first step here, the development of a research idea, is the essence of this chapter and places it in its proper perspective with the whole* (Harbury, 1966).

I present to you a diagram for the practitioner with a complete commitment to a research project. My 30 years of experience have led me to see the process as depicted in the diagram called "The Island of Research," shown in Figure 1.1. Notice that one often begins in the City of Hope and the Jungle of Authority before obtaining the courage to venture nearer the Ocean of Experience. Here the really important hypothesis is generated and the study begins. The rest of this book deals with the study design, data collection, instruments, pretest, and data analysis. In no other chapters, however, are the following important places in an investigator's journey mentioned: the Canyon of Despair; Mount Where-are-we-going?; Data Analysis Jungle; Data Fever-Breeding ground; the Delta of "Dirty" Data; the Wreck Heap of Discarded Hypotheses; the Great Fundless Desert; the tempting Bay of Leisure (administration); and the Bog of Lost Manuscripts. Because of their importance, it is anticipated that many of these topics will be covered in future volumes.

*Level 2* entails participation as a coinvestigator; for example, in large-scale research epidemiological studies such as are sponsored by the National Institutes of Health. Level 2 does not involve making original observations, developing a hypothesis, or securing funding. It does, however, carry responsibility for fiscal integrity, working with coinvestigators and a coordinating committee, being responsible for the day-to-day operation of the data collection, and collaborating with the writing committee. Such participation is also possible with industry-sponsored projects, such as clinical trials with the pharmaceutical industry.

*Level 3* entails participation as a "specialist" or advisor to a project concerning any one of the many parameters described under Level 1. The principal content of this volume provides an excellent example, in discussing how to determine the proper instruments to obtain the best

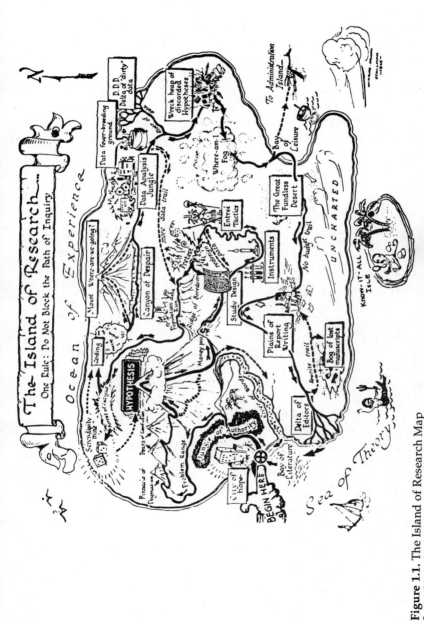

**Figure 1.1.** The Island of Research Map

Source: Map submitted by Dr. Ernest Harbury, Project Director, Program for Urban Health Research (A Study of Stress, Heredity, & Blood Pressure), Dept. of Psychology, The University of Michigan, 405 S. 4th St, Ann Arbor, Michigan. 48103. Permission to reproduce this map granted by American Scientist and the author.

3

results in measuring symptoms, psychosocial factors, quality of life, and so on.

*Level 4* entails participation on a nonfunded basis; for example, as a voluntary observer for the American Cancer Society to report morbidity and mortality data. Stated simply, every practitioner who so chooses can make a significant contribution to the total knowledge base of primary care.

The second area for further clarification concerns the phrase "research in primary care," which carries an ambiguity. Each of its interpretations is laudable and necessary for our discipline, but it is necessary to make a distinction between them, as each requires a different methodological approach. Simply stated, the traditional approach usually has meant looking inward into one's own practice and describing the dynamics of what has been learned in that one practice; the new, expanded approach looks outward into the world at large to interpret what one can observe from the unique observation base of this discipline. *Only you, the primary care physician, have a point of view the specialist does not have.* Research in primary care traditionally has meant studies of the patient population care much in the traditional manner of William Pickles (Pemberton, 1984) and John Fry (1988). Both of these individuals have produced classical examples, such as their research on the prevalence and incidence rates of the common infectious diseases seen in family practice. I myself took this approach within my practice over 30 years ago and am continuing to collect population data in my community in this manner. One of the unique contributions that this approach has afforded me in my practice is the collection of morbidity and mortality rates in black and white population cohorts I have served for a longer period of observation than any other such study. It is allowing me and my collegues to begin to tease out possible etiological factors to help explain the two-fold increase in mortality in blacks over whites.

This expanded interpretation of "research in primary care" reflects a growing awareness of how our truly unique observation base—one that no other discipline has—allows us to study the nature of our species, our responses to the day-to-day environmental challenges we encounter, and our genetic ability to maintain a homeostatic balance between our internal and external milieus.

Paul Nutting (1987), in *Community Oriented Primary Care* (COPC), made a plea to broaden the research spectrum to include the entire community population when he wrote, "A marriage of the principle of epidemiology and the practice of Primary Care (COPC) challenges practitioners to broaden their scope of concern beyond the care of the individual patient" (p. xiii). Dr. J. Bronowski, in *The Ascent of Man* (1973) was saying much the same when he wrote, "There cannot be a philosophy—there cannot even be a decent science, without humanity. For me, the understanding of nature has as its goal the understanding of human nature, and the human condition within nature" (p. 15).

As we all know, humanity and compassion are the essence of our mission. Dr. Jonas Salk was kind enough to invite me to spend several days as his guest at the Salk Institute several years ago, and that visit and experience helped me complete my conceptualization of the truly unique opportunities for research that primary care has to offer. Salk (1972) has said basically the same thing as the others: "For the first time in the evolvement of man, there is the opportunity to understand biology, not only as a science, but also as a basic cultural discipline with unifying potential for the relationship that exists between man and the physical universe, as well as between man and the sciences, arts and humanities" (inside jacket cover). These new opportunities for research are possible in every practice, for those who have the "will."

## Ten Examples From My Office Practice

The following are original observations, made mostly in my own backyard and using no instruments other than my senses of smell, vision, and touch, and the printed word. They are provided to illustrate and substantiate my introductory remarks and also to explain how they made possible an odyssey that has carried me on many exciting adventures (including twice around the world), just as it can for you. Included are examples to illustrate how one can study the world at large from the microcosmos, macrocosmos, and metacosmos (as translated by the philosophers and the poets) in one's own practice.

1.*What constitutes a necessary study site?* Do we necessarily need to live in a city, work in a great university, or have large sums of grant money in order to do good research and make original observations? Is it necessary even to be trained as a research scientist?

*Answer:* Evans County, Georgia, contains no cities. It is a small rural county of 8,000 people, with about 2,500 living in the county seat of Claxton, and is situated 100 miles from the nearest medical school. I have never requested large grant sums, nor have I received special training in epidemiological research. I have had a laboratory in my backyard, however, ever since I received my first chemistry set at around age 10 (and nearly lost my vision on one occasion when a rocket propellent concoction I was making exploded in my face!) I believe anyone can do good research in a rural area, or anywhere else, if he or she has the will. As we all know,

Sir Isaac Newton translated many fundamental laws of nature into mathematical formulae while living in a small cottage in the English countryside—and today his computations are considered so accurate that with very few changes they could have been successfully used for the astronauts' trips to the moon. William Shakespeare had no formal education beyond age 14, yet few have ever lived who even begin to approach his depth and description of the human condition.

I am suggesting that the potential exists for one or more of you to become comparable to these great figures, because I believe the expanded knowledge base of today provides even greater opportunities than existed in former times. Insights today still lie in the eyes of the beholder who dares to *Behold*. This beholder, however, must also have the ambition and determination to follow through to completion any observations and to continue to cultivate a sense of interrelatedness and continuity in all creation. Einstein has reminded us that the most exciting discovery in his entire career was not only to find that rationality and logic exist throughout the universe, but that this was comprehensible by the human mind!

2. *What did a flower bush in my backyard tell me about the past and the future of all living things?*

*Answer:* Two camellia bushes were planted in my yard. Both grew normally and looked identical. Several years later, a garden wall was erected around the house which inadvertently came between the two plants and cut off the sunlight from one. To me, it was a fantastic adventure for the mind and spirit to see this marooned plant make a rational assessment of its environmental problem and select the proper biochemical mechanism for survival, with no neural or brain tissue for synthesizing any thought processes. Only enzymes under genetic control at the cellular level were at work, a process that Rene Dubos (1972) has aptly called "a God within." These genetic mechanisms of survival were later to help me better understand human genetics and its potential—in particular, how sickle-cell anemia in my black patients was helping them resist malaria and yellow fever; and later, the significance of recessive gene mechanisms in general. We no longer see sickle-cell crises in our patients as we did 30 years ago, but recently the United States armed forces have reported that black soldiers who have the sickle-cell trait carry an increased risk (30-40% higher) for sudden death, usually in recruits during strenuous exercise in basic training, than white males, age-adjusted, who do not have the trait. At the Walter Reed Hospital in Washington, where this study was carried out, researchers have no idea what mechanism is involved.

David W. Fisher (1990) recently reported that "more and more evidence accumulates in support of the belief that all cancers have in their pathogenesis, somatic mutations and that very possibly the onco-gene constitutes a natural probe for such a mutation. If this proves true, in whole or in part, and if the human genome is fully sequenced as planned, obviously medical science will have a most powerful possible test for early intervention in the malignant process." For me, this theory has provided another example of a unique opportunity in primary care research: to collect family cohorts and DNA material, either for my own research or to share with geneticists. My practice site has provided a very large cohort (over 200 family members) and has allowed me to share this material with geneticists in many major universities in the United States, Europe, and the National Institutes of Health.

Dr. James Mosley, when asked to describe what genetics meant to him, responded with true sublimity when he wrote, "Genetics is the study which tugs at the veil of fate, permitting man to view, ever after, the mystery of his creation; from the trembling order of his atoms to the 'angels'—sublime or fallen—of his mind; yet it remains the mystery of how a ceaseless generation of uniqueness enshrines the enduring essence of human kind" (Muench, 1989). My translation of this quote is that there is a paradox. In the presence of incredible diversity, the species (or genotype) stays the same. No one knows how or why. The field of genetics offers many great opportunities for research in primary care.

*3. How do 6-million-year-old seashells found in my yard possibly relate to increased cardiovascular disease in Georgia?*

*Answer:* Geologists tell us that 200 million years ago a shifting of the earth's tectonic plates occurred, at which time what is now the continent of Africa pushed into Georgia as far as where presently stand the cities of Columbus, Macon, and Augusta, in the mid-lower half of the state. At the same time, this tremendous force pushed up the Southern Appalachian mountain chain north of Atlanta. Following this, Africa migrated to its present position, and the Atlantic Ocean extended in as far as what is now the middle of the state. The freezing and thawing of the Southern Appalachian Mountains eventually produced a sediment that pushed the sea back to where it is today. Geologists tell us the Atlantic Ocean was in Evans County 6 million years ago with the old seabed 300 to 500 feet below the surface. When I had a well drilled for water in my yard, the drill went into this old seabed. This explained why I was finding seashells. Of interest to me is that apparently, as the sea was pushed back, the wave action eluted certain trace elements from the soil to help create a defined geographical area. This same area has recorded some of the highest death rates in Georgia: It is known as the "stroke belt." It has in the past years reported the highest total mortality rates for stroke and cerebrovascular disease in the United States and one of the highest in the world.

Some of my patients describe their home addresses as on the "Level." This area, which is truly level, is an ancient marine terrace created during the Pleistocene Era more than 2 million years ago, extending down the center of the Florida peninsula. I found that these old seabeds in my county contained major deposits of titanium, an element which, because of its special properties to withstand extremely high temperatures, has made possible the jet engine (and thereby changed human history forever). The Dupont company is mining titanium on this same terrace further south in Florida, and I invited their prospecting team to evaluate the deposits I had found. A two-person prospecting team came with their Geiger counters. We had a wonderful day exploring even though the deposits turned out to be not of commercial quality but were placed on their resources list for use in a national emergency.

How do these same sands relate to my day-to-day practice of medicine? The sands are almost totally devoid of organic material and hence were of little good for use in farming. One could buy this land for $2.00 an acre during the Depression. It became a main source of land to live on, however, and even to try to farm, for almost a fourth of our population. This compounding of many disadvantages created the greatest geographical area for increased disease and its social consequences in my practice: polio, hookworm, other parasitic diseases, malaria, chronic anemia, malnutrition, crime, high school dropout rates, and so on. To me, this situation represented a sad, ironic paradox. I saw abject poverty, yet in the dust underfoot I saw the seeds of change for the world and for unborn generations.

In another example, my neighbor placed 50,000 baby chicks in his chicken house to raise, of which 30,000 promptly died. Other farmers in the area had also experienced the same problem. I went to the University of Georgia's School of Agriculture, and asked: Do any diseases of chickens in South Georgia not exist in North Georgia? The immediate reply was yes: fatty degeneration of the liver, which can easily be corrected by adding selenium to the diet. It was this simple answer that led me to ask the same questions concerning my patients and increased my study of this problem on a worldwide basis. This carried me to the areas known to have low selenium and possible health problem deficiencies—Finland, New Zealand, and China—and increased my studies to include the rest of our own stroke belt, that is, most of South Carolina and the eastern half of North Carolina, which follow the same geographical pattern of increased morbidity and mortality as described for Georgia. I hope by now you can begin to understand the importance of studying interdependencies and how they can relate not only to your own practice but often to the world at large.

4. *What did Georgia's Poet Laureate know 130 years ago about Georgia that we did not know?*

*Answer:* Poets are often said to be 100 years ahead of their time: Sidney Lanier (1900), Poet Laureate of Georgia, was one such person. As mentioned earlier, all cause-mortality rates in South Georgia are much greater than elsewhere. In his "Song of the Chattahoochee," Lanier chose the Chattahoochee River, which provides the boundary line between Georgia and Alabama, to be his "Front" in warning people of the dangers of going into South Georgia. He describes the Southern Appalachian Mountains where this river originates in Habersham and Hall Counties on its course to the sea and has the water weeds, laurel (a bushy plant), ferns, grass, dewberry, and reeds all plead with people to stay in the mountains of North Georgia:

> All down the hills of Habersham
> All through the valleys of Hall
> The rushes cried *abide, abide*
> The willful water weeds *held me thrall,*
> The loving Laurel *turned my tide*
> The ferns and the fonding grass *said stay,*
> The dewberry dipped for to *work delay,*
> And the little reeds sighed *abide, abide*
> Here in the valleys of Hall.

Lanier was also intrigued by the marshes of coastal Georgia and asked, "If I could know, what swimmeth below when the tide comes in on the marvellous Marshes of Glenn?" The University of Georgia now has a marine biology station near there to answer these questions. We now, of course, know that these marshlands are, on a per acre basis, some of the most productive land in the world. They provide a safe haven for young fish to mature and make possible our fishing industry. I see the wisdom of the poets as a bridge between the "pure" scientist and the philosopher's translation of the pure scientist's findings into the human idiom. It is an important link in our humanity.

5. *What did that mosquito that bit me in my yard carry?*

*Answer:* At certain times of the day or year, one is almost bound to get bitten by mosquitoes in my yard. I was interested in "slow viruses" as they may be related to Alzheimer's and other chronic diseases. A thousand of my patients were examined for 11 different virus antibody titers— 11,000 determinations in all. In addition I had 5,000 mosquitoes caught and divided into lots of 50 each. From these samples, 21 different virus antibody titers were determined. Encephlomyocarditis was highest in poor blacks who had no window screens in their homes: In these homes the mosquitoes were so bad at times that I have delivered babies in a cloud of smoke produced by burning rags in a can near the patient.

6.*What did moss on the trees tell me about the air I breathed in my yard?*

*Answer:* Moss on trees draws all of its sustenance from the air and is thus a perfect model to study the quality of the air we breathe. Cadmium is known to cause hypertension through kidney damage and to block selenium needed to help prevent oxidative damage from entering the metabolic pool. Cadmium is used in the manufacturing of automobile tires; therefore, I studied the content of cadmium absorbed in the moss along the highways. Levels were found to be exceedingly high next to a major highway but nonexistent several miles away.

7.*What was the relationship between an oddly shaped hole in a pine tree in my yard, and the safety of sailing ships of old, Beck's sarcoid, the economy of Canada, and the use of tall oil?*

*Answer:* This hole in the pine tree was in one of the few remaining old trees that contain examples of the original method of collecting tar and pitch. These substances were used to prevent leaks in sailing ships and were among the first exportable products from America to England in the early 1600s. The tar and pitch, which are hydrocarbons, have also been implicated etiologically in several significant diseases in my practice; for example, Beck's sarcoid and scleroderma, to mention two.

Some 60 years ago, it was becoming apparent that the 40-year growth cycle for producing wood pulp would not be able to supply the world-wide increasing demands of the paper industry and that the situation would become critical if additional sources were not found. The southern United States slash pine had only a 20-year cycle. An economical method of extracting the tar and pitch from its pulp was finally developed in the mid-1930s and played an important role in shifting a large part of the paper industry to the southern states. This switch has created much pollution in my practice area; in addition, the industry uses millions of gallons of pristine water daily, thereby lowering the water table (some 21 feet at my home) and producing saltwater intrusion along the Georgia coast. On a medical note, the tars extracted from the wood pulp, called tall oil, have been used to reduce serum cholesterol levels: They bind with the cholesterol to prevent its dietary absorption in the gastrointestinal tract. Interdependency: events seemingly so far removed from my office practice, yet so closely related to the diseases I treat, the water I drink, and the air I breathe. *Another example of the expanded primary care research base, that is, to look out at the world through knowledge gained in our offices.*

One additional irony to consider before leaving this subject: Ever-increasing specialization in our society and the medical profession comes at a time when a broad vision has never been more sorely needed to perceive and understand such interrelationships as the smokestacks of the United States killing the forests of Canada, the burning of the Amazon forest of Brazil, the greenhouse effect raising global temperatures, and so on.

8. *What did my family dog teach me as we walked in our yard?*

*Answer:* The extreme intelligence and behavior of Mr. Bo, a dog I had observed from his birth to maturity, led me to study the exciting data accumulated by Dr. John Paul Scott (1978) and many others concerning the transitory "windows" for imprinting. This body of research data helped me understand what I was observing as it was literally being played out by Mr. Bo; that is, every form of life is born with survival traits or instincts, not only for the individual organism, but also for the reproduction and survival of its species as well. These survival traits contain many optional traits that allow the organism to respond specifically to its particular environment. These time exposures or open windows to sample or test the environment are for a specific time period, after which, when closed, will stay closed. The length of exposure is related to the length of the life cycle; that is, bacteria and virus exposure are in terms of minutes—while humans' are in terms of years. Hence, the process is called *neuroplasticity*; that is, nervous tissue that can be molded to form neural reflex patterns that will be used by the organism for the rest of its life. How does this phenomenon relate to humans? It has been said that a human being who experiences only hostility with no love or support for the first 6 months of its life (during the "open window period") is more likely to receive feedback to his or her brain that it cannot trust anyone or anything. These children conclude that they must therefore fend totally for themselves if they are to survive, and will henceforth express only total egoism without regard for others. They take what they want. Such behavior is thought to be, in part, the basis for the criminal mind with its increasing burden on all human society. These "early windows of opportunity" for changing lifelong behavior patterns were worked out in dogs such as Mr. Bo, and have, as one example, greatly improved the quality and number of Seeing Eye dogs for the blind. The neurobiochemists have recently identified much of the actual biochemistry that controls the opening and closing of these "windows." These new findings may even abolish the truth of the old saying, "You can't teach an old dog new tricks"; that is, this new discovery will make possible the ability to continue to learn *readily* into advanced old age with its subsequent improvements in the quality of life for the aging individual.

9. *What has the delivery of 2,000 babies in my practice taught me?*

*Answer:* The first baby I delivered is now 43 years old. To be able to look at 2,000 people's lives, often from as early as 8 weeks after conception to the present, is truly an inspiring privilege, which can suggest many new approaches to improve the human condition. We need to start as soon after conception as possible to prevent malnutrition, fetal alcohol syndrome, the many forms of damage from smoking, AIDS infection, and so on. The need to provide total love and parental support from birth to at least 6 years of age as a minimum are only a few of the things I have learned from this cohort.

10. *How was I able to be one of the first to demonstrate that HDL is higher in blacks than in whites (which may help explain the lower coronary disease rates in blacks)—and accomplish this with only $2,000?*

*Answer:* When electrophoresis equipment first became available in the mid-1950s, I secured a complete set for my office lab. At that time, no one had yet made lipoprotein epidemiological comparisons between blacks and whites. After over 7,000 determinations, I felt secure enough with my findings to submit them for presentation and publication to the American Heart Association and was rejected for both. Now, 32 years later, it is a number one topic—almost everywhere you look. So be prepared, if you are rejected, to wait a few decades for public acceptance. Another point: The big institutions in the 1950s were buying $50,000 ultracentrifuge equipment to study the same problem; my equipment cost $2,000. We both came up with basically the same conclusions. This is not a criticism; it is only to suggest that usually where there is a will, there is a way.

## Conclusions

This chapter has tried to expand your horizons of opportunities for research in primary care by urging you not only to look inward to your practice, but also *outward* to the world. Family physicians have an observation base available to no other discipline: the opportunity to see wholes unseen by the specialist, and to thereby help lift all humankind to higher levels of understanding about disease and "man's inhumanity to man."

Other considerations in this chapter include:

- An illustration of the old adage, "Where there's a will, there's a way."
- An illustration of the need to develop a sense of interrelatedness and continuity in all creation.
- An example from the microcosmic world of genetics in molecular biology.

- An example from the macrocosmic world that illustrates how a shifting of the tectonic plates could, 200 million years later, affect the health of patients in a practice—from global events to individual patients!
- An example from the metacosmic world that illustrates the humanity and compassion provided by the wisdom of the poets and philosophers—these qualities are the very essences of our mission as physicians. It is all there—it is for *you* to behold and bring to fruition.

## References

Bronowski, J. (1973). *The ascent of man.* Boston: Little, Brown.

Dubos, R. (1972). *A God within.* New York: Scribner.

Fisher, D. W. (Ed.). (1990). *Hospital practice, 25,* 51.

Fry, J. (1988). *General practice and primary health care: 1940's-1980's.* London: Nuffield Hospitals Trust.

Harbury, E. (1966). The island of research map. *American Scientist, 54*(4), 470.

Lanier, S. (1900). The song of the Chattahoochee. In E. C. Stedman (Ed.), *An American anthology 1787-1900.* Boston: Houghton-Mifflin.

Muench, K. H. (1989). *Genetic Medicine.* New York: Elsevier.

Nutting, P. A. (1987). *Community-oriented primary care: From principle to practice.* (HRSA Publication No. 1987. HRSA PE86-1).

Pemberton, J. (1984). *Will Pickles of Wensleydale: The life of a country doctor.* Exeter: Royal College of General Practitioners.

Salk, J. (1972). *Man unfolding.* New York: Harper & Row.

Scott, J. P. (1978). *Critical periods.* Stroudsburg, PA: Dowden, Hutchinson & Ross, Inc.

# 2 The Measurement of Outcomes in General Practice

DAVID METCALFE

Because the new paradigm of medicine emphasizes the importance of humane medicine, whole-person care and a patient-centered approach, a strong feeling of vindication exists in the disciplines of primary care at this time.

That is all the more reason to make sure that we are rigorous in our investigations into what we do and how we do it. One very important area for investigation is the *effectiveness* of the care we provide, and for that we must be able to measure the results of what we do: that is, the outcomes of care.

It usually has been safe to assume that the goal of medical care is altruistic and that its objectives, albeit unstated, are to save life, to ameliorate suffering, to improve function, or to protect from disease. Today the complexity of the needs for medical care and the multiplicity of technical interventions available make the measurement of outcomes essential as a basis for rational and ethical choice. As clinicians, we have a duty to examine the effectiveness of the care we provide. It is important that politico-economic constraints are not allowed to distort the process.

This chapter describes the opportunities for outcome measurement in primary care, and the scientific, technical, and administrative problems encountered when applying them.

The essential differences between family practice and the specialties are the breadth of the case mix encountered and the range of the natural history of diseases with which the practitioner is concerned. As the effectiveness of health care systems comes under scrutiny, no argument arises about the necessity of measuring outcome in family practice. In the British National Health Service, every working day, 109,000 inpatients are in care and 151,000 outpatients are seen—and 750,000 consultations occur in general practice. Thus, in terms of volume alone, the effectiveness of primary care is of crucial importance. If we are to measure effectiveness in health care systems, it is at the primary care level that much of the work will have to be done.

Before addressing the problems in doing this work, it will be useful to define some terms.

*Outcomes* are the change in health status that result either from medical interventions or from the deliberate decision not to intervene. They cannot, therefore, be measured unless the intervention is accurately described. The description of the intervention must include its explicit objectives so that the end state can be compared to what was intended and thus any unintended changes identified. The use of the term *health status* as the subject for endpoint assessment conforms to WHO definitions in that it goes beyond the presence or absence of pathophysiology and includes psychological and social well-being.

## Purposes of Outcome Measurement

For four reasons we need to be able to measure outcomes:

1. To be more objective in our assessment of our patients' progress and the effectiveness of our management (and, it has been pointed out, to validate our diagnoses);
2. To be able to compare the effectiveness of one treatment with another;
3. To validate the process criteria developed for clinical audit; and
4. To assess cost effectiveness.

As clinicians, our first concern must be with the first two purposes: More valid and more reliable outcome measures should be everyday tools of the trade. As clinical audit becomes established as a mainstream activity of clinicians rather than merely the concern of quality assurers, we must make sure that process criteria (which are the most tempting to establish and apply) are justified by measurable improvements in outcome.

Quality has three components: *effectiveness* (the extent to which the objectives of care are achieved), *efficiency* (the extent to which resources were conserved in achieving effectiveness), and *acceptability* to the patient. Efficiency can only be assessed when care has been shown to be effective, and cost can only be linked to effectiveness if the latter can be measured. To measure effectiveness, therefore, we need to be able to measure outcomes.

Evaluations based on comparisons of costs of process, regardless of effectiveness, would be very dangerous because administrative measures based only on such data—however attractive to politicians and administrators—would be disastrous.

## Problems of Measurement

Before discussing outcome measurements in detail, I want to address two sorts of problems: those of scientific philosophy, and those of technical application.

### PHILOSOPHICAL PROBLEMS

The philosophy of science is founded on the need for reliability: The scientific understanding of our world must be trustworthy because it influences everything we do. The benchmarks of good science have been generalizability, predictive power, and objectivity.

Faced with uncertainty and dogged by failure (in that all our patients eventually die), the medical profession takes refuge in its scientific basis. It is more comfortable with measurements than with pictures or tunes, and it likes them when they are apparently objective and predictive; for example, laboratory results. It is reassuring to have "hard data," even if they are not the data that are needed to solve the problem. Indeed, the desired objectivity and reliability may be bought at the expense of validity, in the sense that the observations that can be made using such tests may not be directly related to the problem being addressed. This value system systematically underrates the usefulness of personal observation and interpretation, despite the fact that in all the rest of our lives we depend on them! Accordingly, a built-in tension in clinicians exists between the urge to be "scientific" and the habit of relying on training and experience. This anomaly is powerfully explored by Schwarz and Wiggins (1988). Health services research deals largely with interactions between people or between people and such factors as disease and treatment. But all human beings are, by definition, unique and the situations in which they can find themselves almost infinitely variable, so inherent limitations to generalizability occur. While reliability is a desirable quality and very necessary in such areas as causality or comparisons of treatment, it can never be achieved to laboratory standards.

Efforts to "harden" the methodology, for example by using ever bigger populations and ever more sophisticated statistics in an attempt to attain such standards, often impose costs on validity. Schon (1984), in a remarkable paper presented at Harvard, pointed out that while professions are based on what he called the "hard, high ground" of laboratory science, their professionals practice out in much more marshy areas. That is, they have to deal with problems that have not yet got laboratory solutions or for which laboratory solutions will never be found because they cannot be stated in terms that facilitate a laboratory approach. Faced with a difficult problem, professionals tend either to pretend that they are still in the cool clean laboratory, regardless of the multiplicity of unidentified or uncontrollable variables, or to select only those components of the problem that are susceptible to what they see as rigor and leave the rest unaddressed. Schon advocates a third response: learning by reflection on action rather than by the application of the cool, clean laboratory yardstick.

Schwarz and Wiggins (1988), in their chapter in Kerr White's marvelous book *The Task of Medicine*, deploy a rigorous critique of laboratory approaches to human function and feeling. Reason and Rowan (1981), in *Human Inquiry*, point out that you cannot research human behavior as if you were looking at organisms in a petri dish: People are aware of the observer, and the observer reacts as a fellow human being. They maintain that conventional "objectivity" is unobtainable and make a strong case for participant research.

When it comes to validity, scientific inquiry cannot divorce itself from the fact that much of the important information on which clinical decisions are made is not measurable and can only be acquired subjectively. To separate out only those parts of the clinical transaction that can be subjected to "objective," quantified measurement is to lose validity. It could be argued that the consultation between the doctor and the patient is a prime example of participant research, using a small population! We therefore have to maintain a proper sense of proportion in health services research with regard to reliability and objectivity. What we in medicine must not do is to use spurious values to denigrate the wealth of research being undertaken by our colleagues in the behaviorial and social sciences. For as soon as we go beyond simple parameters of physiological, biochemical, or anatomical characteristics into the realms of feelings and social function, it is to these disciplines that we must look for help.

Today, with ideas from the new paradigm at last bridging the Cartesian mind-body chasm, and the emergence of ideas about psychoneuroimmunology beginning to take shape, such cooperation becomes essential. The measurement of outcomes is a good starting place for this, in that it is of immediate usefulness and importance.

## TECHNICAL PROBLEMS

Five problems are to be overcome if outcome measurement is to be generally applicable, valid, and reliable:

1. Differentiating between acute disease treatment and chronic illness management;
2. Establishing explicit objectives (where traditionally the profession has preferred to leave them implicit);
3. Achieving a comprehensive definition of the intervention in those situations in which it is complex;
4. Developing and selecting measurements of physical status, feelings, and function that are valid, reliable, and applicable; and
5. Applying such measures at an appropriate time after the intervention, or in the natural history of the disease.

These issues are discussed in turn below.

### Differentiation Between Disease Treatment and Illness Management

Measurements of outcome must be valid; that is, they must measure real progress toward the goals of care. When these are complex, addressing several needs, several measures of outcome will be needed. For this reason, it is important to differentiate between treatment and management. *Treatment* describes a relatively circumscribed range of technical interventions focused primarily on the pathophysiology: disease-centered care. *Management* describes the range of interventions, of which treatment is just one part, directed to the totality of the patient's ill- health—physical, social, and psychological: patient-centered care.

Disease-centered care is appropriate in inpatient settings, particularly for people with acute illness who are in no position to try to carry out normal social function. On the other hand, in family practice, and particularly in the care of chronic and psychiatric illness, the objectives, and therefore the measurements of outcome, must be management-orientated and person-centered. Perhaps we should adopt the rule that only when patients have little or no autonomy, for example when they are in a hospital, can care be purely disease-centered and its outcomes measured in pathophysiological terms. When patients are autonomous and particularly when they are in their normal environments, care must be person-centered and outcomes measured in terms of health status.

## Objectives of Care

The lack of explicit objectives precludes a rational choice of outcome measures in all but the simplest of cases. If you do not know what the doctor was trying to achieve, how do you know what to measure? Without explicit and agreed-on objectives, judgments could be made on the wrong parameters. Up to now, setting explicit objectives for medical care has not been part of the culture (even though Weed [1969] was advocating it back in the sixties). Presumably this has been because, until comparatively recently, the main medical task has been the care of acute infectious disease or trauma, in which the objectives are so obvious that they do not need to be made explicit. Now, with chronic disease control and the care of old people with multisystem failure as the largest part of our work, such failure to set objectives both makes us vulnerable to providing poor care and frustrates efforts to evaluate it. For example, if I fail to set explicit objectives for the care of a patient with rheumatoid arthritis, I will end up titrating treatment against pain and may well fail to protect the patient from disability. If, on the other hand, I write down "Control pain, prevent ulnar deviation and flexion deformities of the fingers," or better still, "Control pain, keep ESR below 20, maintain ability to type and knit," I not only have a comprehensive agenda for each consultation, but three parameters on which to judge my effectiveness.

## Defining and Describing the Intervention

In acute illness or in the inpatient episodes of a chronic disease, the interventions are discrete and relatively simple because they mostly have short-term goals. Analysis of office consultations has revealed that intervention is a mixture of contributions, all of which are valued by patients and which therefore might all be expected to contribute to improved health status. These include taking the patient seriously, explaining and reassuring, agreeing to goals and plans, supporting or training lay caregivers, and prescribing or referring for specific treatment. All of these may have an appreciable effect on the patient's subsequent well-being: Which one did the most good?

## Developing an Adequate Range of Measuring Tools

Health is broader than the absence of disease: The concept also includes functional capacity and feelings. General practice care is directed at all components of health, using different sorts of interventions for each. Many components of physical status are amenable to measurement: TSH, peak flow, blood pressure, or joint mobility, for example. Imaging and endoscopy are available for the inspection of lesions. These are comfortably "scientific" and "objective," and we set great store by them, but they are only part of the sick person's global health status. Symptom relief is always an important objective but must be assessed subjectively by the patient. Moreover, it is vulnerable to mood changes, which may themselves be the result of confounding variables (such as difficulty in getting an appointment). People's pain thresholds vary with mood. Activities of Daily Living measures (Katz, Ford, Moskowitz, Jackson, & Jaffe, 1963) are more objective, to the extent that they are assessed by an observer rather than the patient. They still depend, however, on that observer's subjective judgment of the extent to which the patient's functions conform to the descriptions in the scales. Moreover, functional capacity has been shown to be affected by other components of the illness, such as the amount of pain being experienced at the time of measurement.

Subtler subjective changes, such as self-image and self-confidence, are important components of well-being and therefore are also goals of good comprehensive care. Some diseases and some treatments affect body image too, with marked effects on well-being: for example, acne and obesity; amputation and mastectomy. All of these need sensitive and sophisticated measures if they are to be evaluated.

The plethora of scales for measuring personal and social function and feelings, and the extensive literature assessing their validity and reliability, attest to the fact that this is neither simple nor easy. Chapters 10, 11, and 12 deal with such scales, and Chapters 5 and 6 deal with the assessment of reliability and validity. Those measures that seem to stand up best to evaluation of their performance seem to require fairly expert administration by workers with trained social science skills and are therefore suitable for research but of limited applicability by untrained and busy clinicians.

## Deciding When to Measure Outcome

For inpatient care, discharge or attendance at a follow-up clinic offers easy and sensible endpoints at which to assess the outcome. Except in simple acute conditions, however, this may not be the appropriate moment in the natural history of the illness to judge the effectiveness of the care provided. Indeed, one of the objectives of care may merely be to slow down the expected progression of the disease; to alter the trend. To measure health status at one point in time in a relapsing condition like multiple sclerosis would also produce invalid results. Prudence dictates as long an interval as possible between the intervention and the outcome measurement, to give the maximum time for benefit to accrue and for unlooked-for events to occur. The longer it is left, however, the more vulnerable is the connection between intervention and outcome to intervening variables.

## Tasks in Primary Medical Care

With these difficulties in mind, I would now like to discuss the different tasks we do in general practice in terms of their objectives and the outcome measures that will be needed.

General practitioners undertake the following main tasks to meet the needs of their patient populations:

- Primary and secondary prevention (screening and case finding)
- Exclusion of serious illness
- Acute disease care
- Chronic illness care
- Care of psychiatric illness
- Terminal care

This list provides a framework for developing, choosing, and applying outcome measures.

### Prevention

*Objectives:* Primary prevention by removal or neutralization of causal factors. Secondary prevention by early diagnosis (where earlier means better).

*Outcome measures:* Primary: incidence in population. Secondary: death rate or serious complication rate in population.

The outcomes of primary preventive care are not measurable in individuals because they are nonevents! They are only measurable in terms of the reduced incidence of the index disease in the populations concerned (which may have to be large if the condition is relatively rare). Because of this, a tendency exists to measure intermediate outcomes such as population coverage, which is really a process variable. Also, sometimes what is being measured is not really the desired outcome itself: for example, a reduction in cholesterol levels in a population is not the actual goal; the desired outcome is a reduction in coronary deaths. When only intermediate or surrogate outcomes are available, it is important to be open about this. The use of intermediate outcomes for assessment of cost effectiveness is probably invalid because of the problem of differentiating base and marginal costs, so the cost of coverage is only crudely proportional to the cost of saving each case. Moreover, the use of coverage as an outcome measure precludes the chance of investigating some unwanted effects of screening that are costs to the patient: anxiety about needing the tests, anxiety when waiting for the results, and the trauma of false positives.

### Exclusion of Serious Illness

*Objective:* Reliable (i.e., safe) reassurance.

*Outcome measures:* Absence of subsequent disease for which presenting complaint could have been a harbinger; subjective reduction in anxiety in the patient (where anxiety has been the reason for presentation).

A very large proportion of new presentations to family practitioners is for reassurance: problems that, although with hindsight and expertise we may regard as "trivial," were worrying enough to the patient to motivate a visit. Exclusion of serious illness (perhaps the most important clinical task, the real "gatekeeper" role) requires proper history taking, examination, and sometimes investigation, as a basis for reliable reassurance. This is a major intervention in itself: It is important to stress that exclusion is usually more intellectually challenging than most diagnosis, which is mainly a matter of pattern recognition. Exclusion also has as its outcome a nonevent: The illness that the patient explicitly or implicitly feared is not present and does not supervene. The desired outcome is the improvement in health that comes from transferring status from worried well to unworried well, but since the grateful patient disappears, this is difficult to measure! Follow-up audits could reveal failure by identifying people who had had their nonmedical conditions medicalized (false positives) and those in whom serious illness that could have been spotted has supervened (false negatives).

### Acute Physical Illness or Trauma

*Objectives:* Removal or correction of disease process; repair of trauma, restoration of function.

*Outcome measures:* Presence or absence of pathology; recovery or nonrecovery of function.

Acute illness or trauma is managed by treatment and advice, possibly with support from allied professions or by referral to specialist care. In the short-term the objectives are simple and are seldom made explicit:

The care is disease-centered and is usually evaluated by measurement of physical parameters or by simple assessment of physical capability. Restoration of function, however, particularly after the repair of trauma, depends not only on physical parameters but on psychological (for example, self-confidence and body image) and social (for example, employment opportunities) ones as well.

### Chronic Physical Illness

*Objectives:* Control of disease process; reduction of subjective distress; restoration, or maintenance, of function.

*Outcome measures:* Objective measures of pathophysiology; subjective measure of experience; objective measures of function.

The pathophysiology of chronic disease dictates the objectives in terms of the reversal, control, or slowing down of the disease process. These interventions are those of technical medicine, and outcomes are measured in terms of the progress of the disease process. But distress, including loss of self-image or even of acceptable body image, and frustration with disability must be identified and reduced by symptom control, counseling, and support (including support for caregivers). The outcome of these interventions can be measured by symptom scores, health diaries, or general scales such as the Nottingham Health Profile or the Sickness Impact Profile, and, importantly, in interviews with caregivers.

Objectives in the domain of function are directed to recovery or maintenance of self-care, occupational and household capability, and social interaction. Interventions will include nursing, the provision of appliances, rehousing, and training, as well as specific therapies. The outcomes must be measured by observers rating the patients' behavior and capabilities in these fields.

### CARE OF PSYCHIATRIC ILLNESSES

Psychological disease varies from florid psychosis to normal reactions to social stress, and the whole spectrum is seen in general practice.

### Psychosis

*Objectives:* Protection from self harm; reduction of distress; support for family caregivers.

*Outcome measurements:* Self-harm happens or does not happen; recorded by patients (but patients' illness may make them unreliable witnesses);

family caregivers' expression of satisfaction with the extent to which their perceived needs were met.

At the psychotic end of the spectrum, the illnesses conform to the pattern of relapsing chronic physical diseases but without easily measured parameters of status or progress. With so little understanding of the nature of these diseases, care in the acute phase is essentially a holding operation, using drugs and surveillance, and in the chronic phases is designed to maintain calm while restoring social function. Family and other caregivers are a particularly important resource but also have needs for support themselves if not downright care. Thus their function and feelings should also be the subject of outcome measurement if the psychotic patient's care is really being evaluated. The difficulty in applying such instruments in these cases is, of course, that the very nature of the illness makes the principal witness unreliable. Nevertheless, a variety of interview schedules and behaviorial rating scales are in use that have been shown to have acceptable reliability. The main problem is with validity; considerable argument arises about whether these instruments truly measure what is going on in the patient's head.

### Neurosis

*Objectives:* Reduction of distress; restoration of self-management; improvement of self-image.

*Outcome measurements*: Distress recorded by patient; personal and social function measurement; self-image as assessed by observer.

At the emotional dysfunction end of the spectrum, the natural history is much less predictable and the objectives for care therefore fairly pragmatic. Interview schedules and standardized psychiatric questionnaires, such as the General Health Questionnaire (Goldberg, 1972), are useful in this area—particularly in depression, which is a more clear-cut entity. These are, however, mainly assessments of symptoms and feelings rather than function, which can still be considerably disturbed, and it is important to measure that too.

### Terminal Illness

*Objectives:* Symptom control; maintenance of function; achievement of acceptance (peace of mind).

*Outcome measures:* Caregiver or professional observers; assessment of daily living/social function by patient and caregivers; assessment of peace of mind by patient and caregivers.

Terminal illness requires a balance of interventions with objectives that include symptom control, maintenance of personal and social function, and the achievement of acceptance of impending death. Here the difficulty is that the most sensitive indicator of effectiveness of care is the evidence of the patients themselves, but most doctors are hesitant to submit their dying patients to assessments of symptoms, function, and feelings, particularly before they had come to terms with the fact that they were dying. Relatives too are unlikely to be very objective, having their own needs. Sensitive and acceptable studies have been done by social scientists on a research basis, and spending unhurried time with a dying patient is the most valuable form of assessment. It would be difficult, however, to incorporate outcome measures routinely into terminal care.

## Five Questions When Evaluating Primary Care

Whether we are seeking to evaluate the effectiveness of a single doctor's care or a whole specialty, or the care provided in one district or in a whole system, we are faced with huge problems of volume and variety. As mentioned, in the U.K. 750,000 GP-patient encounters occur every day, covering all kinds of diseases, at every stage in the natural history of those diseases, and involving interactions (such as the exclusion of serious illness) that are not describable by conventional classification systems such as the ICD-9. It is patently impossible to apply outcome measures on this scale, so we must make choices. The choices we make are vitally important because the process of assessment of effectiveness will itself change behavior, independently of the changes made in incorporating the findings into clinical practice and its politico-administrative management. These choices include five questions:

1. Which of the clinical activities described should be evaluated, whether internally or externally? (And if any should not be evaluated, why should they be undertaken at all?)
2. How many examples of each type of clinical activity should be subjected to outcome measurement, and which ones? Would a "tracer" condition be a reliable indicator of effectiveness in other, similar clinical activities?
3. How often should such measurements be made, especially in view of the problems of intervening variables and of identifying appropriate times in the natural history?

4. By whom should the instruments be applied: the GPs, or appropriately trained social scientists? Equally, by whom should the scores be analyzed, and using what skills?

5. What resources from within or without the practice should be dedicated to outcome measurement, and what costs are containable?

The temptation, of course, is to develop outcome measurements only for easily identified and "important" interventions and not for the rest of the protean activities of the family practitioner. To succumb to this, however, would not only forfeit the chance of examining the overall effectiveness of the primary care sector but might actually skew the pattern of care provided. It is conceivable that some doctors would begin to concentrate their efforts on conditions amenable to outcome measurement, while others might take avoiding action by selective referral. This might depend on their clinical self-confidence. If outcome measures are to be applied externally to evaluate general practice, the application of only those instruments from bioscience that are used to measure physical status will result in a corresponding bias in the way GPs set their objectives and provide care. Politico-economic pressures for a "quick fix" could have serious effects on the sensitivity and comprehensiveness of care.

## Conclusion

Family practice needs to be able to measure outcomes just as much as the other clinical disciplines and for the same reasons. The wide variety of tasks that characterize family practice and the multiplicity of the domains in which improvement is attempted necessitate the development of a correspondingly wide range of measuring instruments if validity is to be achieved.

Books like this one are an essential step forward. They facilitate productive interaction between social, behaviorial, and clinical scientists and diminish the negative feelings that often exist between them. Tension does exist between research *in* and research *on* family practice (I do not like to feel, in my clinical work, that I am squirming about on somebody's petri dish). But if we see the endeavor as a two-circle Venn diagram, one circle being the activities of clinicians and the other circle being the activities of the social and behaviorial scientists, it is from the overlap area that a grounded theory will emerge. Here I would like to make a plea about the qualitative-quantitative argument, for which I feel some responsibility, since in my address to the Tenth Annual Meeting of the North American Primary Care Research Group I asked for a shift from digital to analog. Quantitative and qualitative *methodologies* can be seen as fixed points along a spectrum—researchers using appropriate tools must be able and prepared to move about on that spectrum. Here they could take a leaf from the notebooks of clinicians who, in one consultation, can move between millimolecular weights of trace elements to social chat about the patient's family in what, in my own consultations, can seem to be almost Brownian movement!

Medicine is a fine endeavor, a many splendored thing. We owe it to ourselves, to those who give us a mandate to care for them, and to those whom we teach who will follow us, to be rigorous in our assessment of what we achieve.

## References

Goldberg, D. P. (1972). *The detection of psychiatric illness by questionaire.* Oxford, UK: Oxford University Press.

Katz, S., Ford, A. B., Moskowitz, R. W., Jackson, B. A., & Jaffe, M. W. (1963). Studies of illness in the aged, index of ADL: A standardized measure of biological and psychosocial function. *Journal of the American Medical Association, 185,* 914-919.

Reason, P., & Rowan, J. (Eds.). (1981). *Human inquiry: A sourcebook of new paradigm research* (pp. 137-171). Chichester: John Wiley.

Schon, D. A. (1984). *The crisis of professional knowledge in the pursuit of an epistemology of practice.* Paper presented at Harvard Business School, 75th Anniversary Colloquium on Teaching by the Case Method, Cambridge, MA.

Schwarz, M. A., & Wiggins, O. P. (1988). Scientific and humanistic medicine: A theory of clinical methods. In K. L. White (Ed.), *The task of medicine: Dialogue at Wickenburg* (pp. 18-19). Menlo Park, CA: Henry J. Kaiser Family Foundation.

Weed, L. (1969). *The medical record, medical education and patient care: The problem-oriented record as a basic tool.* Cleveland, OH: Case Western University Press.

# PART ONE

# BASIC CONCEPTS

## 3 The Clinician in Research: Identifying Questions and Observing

MARTIN J. BASS

As clinicians, we are in a position to play a significant role in primary care research. We can fulfill two particular functions. The first is in identifying researchable questions; the second is as an observer and a measuring instrument.

Both advantages and disadvantages exist to clinicians being involved in research, and these are very closely intertwined. First, the physician is by definition present at all physician-patient contacts but has the main objective of attending to the patient's clinical problems. Thus any research measure that the clinician is interested in must be easily incorporated into the process of clinical care. It must not detract from this care or demand too much time or alter the doctor-patient relationship; if it does, it will not be completed. Second, clinicians are highly trained and are in a position to provide a great deal of complex data; however, this training is not always a guarantee against high individual variability in measurement. For research results to be meaningful, each physician must learn to measure the factor under study—whether blood pressure or the degree of anxiety—in exactly the same manner. Third, to purchase a clinician's time to undertake research can be costly. If the clinician is intimately involved in the research project, however, his or her labor is often provided as part of the clinical care. This enables physicians to undertake research with little extra cost.

## Identifying Researchable Questions

In the course of caring for patients, the frontline practitioner becomes aware of many aspects of disease and illness that do not appear in textbooks, and may develop hypotheses and explanations that both satisfy the situation of the moment and reflect the context of the patient's environment. To illustrate, I was recently troubled by the following three interactions that occurred in my clinical practice:

- A 90-year-old patient had a long history of chronic obstructive lung disease. The day her son went on a well-deserved and long-overdue holiday, she suffered a respiratory arrest. There seemed to be no precipitant other than her son's departure. Reviewing the literature, I could not find any reported cases of acute stress as a cause of respiratory arrest in patients with chronic respiratory disease; however, I wondered: Could this be what happened?

- An elderly patient was brought to the emergency department by her exhausted relatives, who reported that she had fallen and that they could no longer care for her. I wondered: If I been more alert before the fall, could I have identified that the relatives were reaching the end of their tether and prevented this crisis?

- A young woman presented with three small venereal warts. They responded well to podophyllin, but I was left wondering: Does this patient have a greater risk of developing carcinoma of the cervix by virtue of the papilloma virus present? Should I be doing cervical screening more frequently than I normally would?

The preceding three questions all arose from my clinical encounters and the reflections that occurred during and after those contacts, and each seemed to me to be eminently researchable and worthy of pursuit. While not of the significance and depth of the questions outlined by Hames in Chapter 1, they do bear a resemblance in that they too arise from clinical situations. Dr. Hames has given us some excellent examples of the clinician's ability to identify areas worthy of pursuit and then to help formulate a research question, such as his observing a pattern of heart attacks in patients from the lowlands, and wondering whether any connection existed with the fact that the soil there was lacking in an essential element. While few of us will have the ability to pose such a broad range of questions, we can all learn from our own experiences.

A clinician can identify important questions in several ways. The first, as seen by my examples and those of Hames, is to look at cases that trouble you and to see whether the answers are available from standard sources. If they are not, then you probably have identified a researchable question. (Another excellent example of this is the work of Dr. K. B. Thomas [1987], who hypothesized that if a physician is positive about a therapy, that therapy will be more effective; and then elegantly showed this in a randomized trial.)

A second approach to identifying important research questions is to listen to your patients. A recent example of this is seen in the work of Dr. J. Southern and colleagues (Southern, Smith, & Palmer, 1990). In investigating an outbreak of diarrhea in children in which campylobacter was implicated, these clinicians were stimulated to a specific research question by a mother who wondered if her son's diarrhea could have had anything to do with the fact that his milk bottle had been attacked by magpies a couple of days earlier. A subsequent case control study in fact showed a strong relationship between bird attacks on milk bottles and the development of diarrhea. Similarly, in a study in which I was pursuing prognostic factors in patients who present with headache (Headache Study Group, 1986), one physician proposed the hypothesis that patients would be more likely to improve if the doctor liked them. This observation had come from a patient's report that this physician had been instrumental in helping resolve her headache because he seemed to care. This hypothesis, which was supported by the results, appeared to be based on the fact that patients who are liked are given a greater opportunity to discuss their headaches and the problems surrounding them.

The sorts of questions that clinicians generate from their interactions with patients come, as we have seen, from both within the physician and from listening to the patient. Such questions can only be generated by clinicians in the field; full-time researchers or scientists removed from the clinical setting will not identify them.

## The Clinician As Observer

As physicians, we are underutilized tools in research. We can play a key role in gathering the traditional objective measures of medical practice and research, such as blood pressure, hemoglobin, and weight. But equally important can be our role in gathering subjective data based on our impressions and feelings.

I have identified five sources of physician-derived data: (a) questions, (b) devices, (c) clinical observation, (d) clinical judgment, and (e) self-reflection.

## Physician-Derived Data

1. *Questions.* In a research study, the questions the physician asks of patients could, in many cases, be gathered by questionnaires or in interviews by

research personnel. The advantage of having the clinician do the asking personally is that most of the data are required in any case for clinical care (the questions most often posed are related to duration of the problem, onset, accompanying features, relieving features, and other items of medical and family history). Thus the research is simply incorporated into the usual process of care and in fact may assist the physician in obtaining an orderly history of the problem for clinical purposes.

2. *Devices.* The technological devices typically used in clinical care (e.g., sphygmomanometer, urine protein dipstick, glucometer, peak flow meter) can also be important sources of data for research studies. The instruments themselves obviously require calibration and determination of their accuracy; equally important, however, is the calibration of the observer who is using them. This requires training to ensure reliable, accurate, readings and standard approaches to use. The lack of standardization and accuracy of clinicians' measurements was identified as a problem many years ago by Bourne (1931), who made recommendations for improvements. This theme has been echoed more recently by Feinstein (1987) and Koran (1975) and is essential to the conduct of good clinical research.

3. *Clinical observation.* The third area of physician-derived data is that of clinical observation, whereby clinicians use their own senses to obtain data. Examples of this type of data could be the determinations of sinus tenderness, swelling of the ankles, or heart murmur; in the same category but in a totally different vein are observations on depression, anxiety, and mood in general. As with data obtained with devices, the physician-observer must adhere to standards and have a clear definition of what is being measured. It is important that one's observations be reliable and accurate. This is best assessed by being observed by peers as one works through a protocol with a patient. If this assessment is being carried out in a workshop, then groups of clinicians can compare their differences, discuss any discrepancies, and decide on approaches to ensure a standard result. In addition, in any long-term study it is important to check that the instrument—in this case the physician—*maintains* accuracy.

4. *Clinical judgment.* In the preceding three categories a trained observer could take on the role of the physician; however, in the area of clinical judgment the physician is irreplaceable. Clinical judgment implies making use of one's experience and knowledge base, as well as one's knowledge of the particular patient, to summarize all the information obtained and make a "best decision," which becomes part of the data set. An example of this would be a judgment about whether a particular factor is operating as a cause of a patient's problem—say, is anxiety a contributing cause to this patient's headache? Clearly this approach brings a large complexity of interacting patterns to bear. It uses the *experience* of the clinician for the benefit of the research—an untapped area in primary care research.

5. *Self-reflection*. In the fifth type of measure, the physician truly acts as a measuring instrument: considering his or her own *feelings* about an interaction and reporting them to become part of the data set. This is an important factor in Balint's (1955) approach to the patient but has rarely been used in prognostic studies. The use of self-reflection gives value to subjective data. While this use may cause concern for those trained in disease epidemiology, it reflects the distinctive characteristics of family practice, in which the patient is the focus of care and often the doctor is the main therapy. Thus research into doctor-patient interactions and outcomes of care must of necessity involve subjective measures such as those determined by self-reflection and clinical judgment.

## An Illustration

To illustrate the preceding five types of data that clinicians can collect, the remainder of this chapter describes a recent study conducted at the University of Western Ontario. This study entailed recruiting physicians as participant/observers.

The study started by involving participants in the choice of the topic to be examined. All part-time clinical teachers in the department were asked whether they would be interested in looking at the natural history of common symptoms seen in practice, and those who attended an organizational meeting selected headache as being of greater interest than chest pain, fatigue, back pain, or dizziness. They were then asked to suggest factors that they felt were predictive of outcome in their headache patients; these factors were incorporated into the study.

Finally, these physicians were responsible for personally obtaining many of the study measures, which spanned all five types of data listed above. They were instructed to ask their patients whether their headache was a major problem and to describe its duration and characteristics, as well as factors that worsened or relieved it (*questions*). They were asked to record diastolic blood pressure using calibrated sphygmomanometers, measuring it precisely at the cessation of sound with the cuff applied 2 cm above the elbow (*devices*). They were asked to record two types of *clinical observations*: tenderness of the frontal sinuses, and the degree of anger, sadness, and depression exhibited by the patient. For the first, they were instructed to tap over the supraorbital notch to determine the degree of tenderness elicited; this procedure was explained, and each physician's technique was observed in a practice session to ensure uniformity and reliability. Reliability of the second measure was assessed by using an actor whose mood was scored independently by each participant; the results were compared and discussed, and then the procedure was repeated until everyone agreed on the "patient's" presentation. They were asked to tell, in their best judgment, whether anxiety was a cause of any of their patients' headaches (*clinical judgment*). Finally, they were asked to identify their feelings toward each patient at the end of the first visit (*self-reflection*) by answering the question, "How do you feel about this patient?" on a 5-point scale ranging from *Like* to *Dislike*. This question was completed for all patients enrolled in the study, and a wide variation occurred in responses. While it was not possible to check the validity of clinical judgments or feelings toward the patient, it was checked that all participants had a good understanding of what they were asked to record, and they were monitored during the study, being asked specifically about these items.

In this longitudinal study, which continued over 1 year, the data described above were only one part of a data collection that also involved patient-completed questionnaires and interviews by research staff. The final results illustrate the value of the physician-derived measures. The first question looked at was: "What factors on the first visit predict a headache with an organic cause?" The most powerful predictor turned out to be the physician's clinical judgment on the first visit that anxiety was not a contributing factor; the second predictor was the degree of tenderness of the frontal sinuses, as measured by the physician. Another important question was: "What are the predictors of who will do poorly at 1 year?" (A "poor" outcome was defined here as being unable to function for 1 or more days in the month preceding the 12-month follow-up.) In descending order of predictive power were three patient-reported factors: severe pain, the presence of prodromal vomiting, and the absence of a second type of headache. In fourth place, and statistically significant, was the physician-derived self-reflective measure: the degree to which the patient was liked by the doctor on the first visit. Patients not liked were 4.1 times as likely to continue to have problems with their headache at 1 year as those whom the physician did like.

## Conclusion

As primary care research moves more into the areas of doctor-patient communication and interaction and outcome measures, clinician-derived data grow in importance. Research that embodies only such traditional objective measures as demographic data, laboratory tests, drugs prescribed, or scores on anxiety and depression scales may not give us the answers or insights we seek. I want to emphasize the value to physicians of using a readily available, very sensitive instrument for office-based research

—oneself. This instrument is not without flaws: it can be strong willed, have biases, and lack objectivity—but it can also be responsive, flexible, and add the richness of insight to an inquiry.

## References

Balint, M. (1955). *The doctor, his patient, and the illness*. (2nd ed.) London: Pitman Medical.

Bourne, G. (1931). *An introduction to medical history and case taking*. Edinburgh: E & S Livingstone.

Feinstein, A. R. (1987). *Clinimetrics*. New Haven, CT: Yale University.

Headache Study Group of the University of Western Ontario. (1986). Predictors of outcome in headache patients presenting to family physicians: A one-year prospective study. *Headache, 26*, 285-295.

Koran, L. (1975). The reliability of clinical methods, data, and judgements. *New England Journal of Medicine, 293*, 642-646.

Southern, J. P., Smith, R. M. M., & Palmer, S. R. (1990). Bird attack on milk bottles: Possible mode of transmissions of *Campylobacter jejuni* to man. *Lancet, 336*, 1425-1427.

Thomas, K. B. (1987). General practice consultations: Is there any point in being positive? *British Medical Journal, 294*, 1200-1202.

# 4 The International Classification of Primary Care: Health Information for the Future

MAURICE WOOD

The International Classification of Primary Care (ICPC), prepared by the ICPC Working Party and edited by Henk Lamberts and Maurice Wood (1987), breaks new ground in the work of classification. For the first time, using a single classification, health care providers can classify three important elements of the health care encounter: Reason for Encounter (RFE), diagnoses or problems, and the process of care. These three elements may be used separately or concurrently.

## Background

Information systems and health statistics deal with data that have been ordered and have a name, and hence can be counted. What has no name cannot be counted and consequently has no impact; what has an incorrect or incomplete name leads, when counted, to irrelevant data prohibiting practical use or even a sensible interpretation. Ample support exists for the need for a "classification system which allows a shift in the orientation of health information systems and of health services research towards the identification and collection of episode-oriented data" (Lamberts & Wood, 1987, p. 01).

One of the first signs of a change in the orientation of health information systems was the implementation of sentinel practices, which agree to collect data according to standardized rules, a strategy that originated in England in 1968 (Lamberts & Schade, 1988). Since 1970 a network of sentinel practices involving 45 general practitioners has functioned in

The Netherlands, serving about 1% of the population. The idea of gaining insight into the occurrence of certain diseases and their trends over periods of time with the help of data from general practice has occurred in other countries as well. In the United States and Canada, the Ambulatory Sentinel Practice Network has been established (Green et al., 1984), while Australia, Belgium, Canada, Great Britain, Israel, The Netherlands, New Zealand, Switzerland, and the United States cooperate in the International Primary Care Network (ICPN).

Family physicians who do not choose to join a sentinel system can collect comprehensive data on all morbidity presented to them over a long period, such as 1 year. Compared to official notification systems, which often result in incomplete data, continuous clinical information from family practice provides far more reliable data on the incidence of common diseases (Lamberts, 1984; Lamberts, Brouwer, Groen, & Huisman, 1987; Royal College of General Practitioners, 1975). In family practice settings, with known numerators and denominators, data from direct surveillance of clinical information allows extrapolation to national populations for infectious diseases, such as hepatitis A, measles, gonorrhea, and infectious gastroenteritis. Lamberts and Schade (1988), in The Netherlands, have used such data in association with multiplier factors to "correct" official prevalence figures for such conditions.

Family physicians have thus proved able to provide information quickly on shifts in patterns, as, for example, on the disappearance of measles, the extent of influenza epidemics, or the recurrence of whooping cough. The emphasis on the distribution of infectious diseases has been succeeded by attention to noninfectious diseases (for example "lifestyle diseases") and to the potential for prevention of these (National Centre for Health Services, 1985). In addition, the need for information on such problems as contraception, abortion, sports injuries, diabetes, depression, suicidal behavior, and the use of tranquilizers is growing. Morbidity data from general practitioners form an essential link in the chain of sources of information necessary for health statistics. In most countries, however, this chain provides a prevalence-oriented epidemiology, based on the use of the ninth revision of ICD (World Health Organization, 1977). The interpretation of the differences in prevalence, both within and between the links of the chain, is often unsatisfactory.

The analysis of diagnosis-related information from family physicians over the years has led to two conclusions:

1. Numerator problems—the quality of the classifications itself—tend to be underestimated, while denominator problems—the sex/age composition of the population for which incidences and prevalences are calcu-

lated—tend to be overestimated. Lack of definitions for the use of diagnostic terms, and even more seriously, lack of understanding of the relation between the patient's demand for care and the doctor's diagnostic interpretation, limit the interpretation of clinical data (White, 1985).

2. Encounter-based diagnostic information is insufficient for the interpretation of large variations in prevalence of disease and in the utilization of health care, both within and between the links in the information chain (Kilpatrick & Boyle, 1984).

The understanding of the differences in clinical judgment among general practitioners and specialists when they treat patients with such diseases as diabetes, hypertension, depression, or chronic respiratory disease is limited because of the lack of sufficient knowledge of the course over time ("natural history") of these diseases, systematically collected and analyzed on the basis of complete episodes of care. This also applies when assessing the quality and appropriateness of medical care as it is provided during each phase of an episode because the relationship between the demands of the patient, the diagnostic interpretation by the physician, and the medical intervention that is the consequence of both is not clear.

## A New Perspective

Two central issues in family practice specify its professional frame of reference:

1. All patients in the practice can present all problems at all times.
2. Family physicians are responsible for continuity of care, not only conceptually but also factually and personally.

Five important elements of family practice can be identified:

1. Good relationships with patients are necessary in order to allow a very open, broad, and continuous access.
2. Family physicians play an important role in labeling health problems, thus legitimizing medical interventions.
3. Family physicians deal with families as units of care instead of just as individuals, again supporting both accessibility and continuity.
4. Looking at the practice as a population, preventive interventions are significant in the overall goals of family medicine. The setting of family

practice allows screening and preventive interventions with patients attending for other reasons.

5. Long-standing relations with patients are a reality in family practice, as is balancing the values in medicine and in society with the patient's preferences. Therefore the patient and the doctor estimate the utility of specific interventions in light of the patient's particular circumstances.

## Minimum Basic Data Set

In any practice a good age/sex register and reliable patient identifiers are essential parts of an administrative minimal basic data set (MBDS). Internationally, different systems deal with very different administrative burdens (e.g., reimbursement, quality assessment). In an ideal world, standards would be established for

- Patient identification, preferably consisting of sex, date of birth, and initials
- Identification of family and/or address
- A method to identify which patients are also in specialist care
- The structure of the patient data base to support screening and preventive interventions
- A problem list with important chronic medical conditions that have to be monitored over time
- A classification to be used with the MBDS

A variety of other options can be added, such as word processing for prescription and referral letters, reimbursement claims, test ordering, and so on. Also, in an ideal world the system can be used to communicate with other information systems and to gain access to stores with Echo and X-ray images, ECGs, and so on.

A separate problem, much farther down the road, is the restructuring and subsequent computerization of the patient's record.

## Prevalence

Another important aspect in family practice is the frequency distribution of diseases. To illustrate this, steps in the frequency distribution of diseases (prevalence) can be established in a series as follows:

- 5 or more cases of a disease per 1,000 persons per year
- 1 to 5 cases of a disease per 1,000 persons per year

- 0.5 to 1.0 cases of a disease per 1,000 persons per year
- less than 0.5 cases of a disease per 1,000 persons per year

In most European countries general practitioners deal with about 250 different diseases with a prevalence of more than 5 per 1,000 persons per year and with another 500 entities that have a prevalence between 1 and 5. With each prevalence step the number of diagnoses included is estimated to double. For instance, approximately 4,000 different diagnoses occur less than once per 100,000 persons per year.

It is evident that the role of specialists, subspecialists, and sub-sub-specialists is most appropriate for, and in the diagnostic sense best defined in, the prevalence areas below 1 per 1,000, 1 per 100,000, and 1 per 1,000,000 persons per year. Family physicians acting as gatekeepers help sub-sub-specialists see patients with relatively high probabilities of suffering from a seldom-occurring disease.

In addition to the frequency aspect, diagnostic considerations in family practice often differ from those of specialists. Here the negative predictive value—that a certain disease is *not* the cause of the patient's problem—is sometimes more important than the positive predictive value— for which a disease *is* diagnosed with a high degree of certainty. Another difference is that in family practice uncertainty exists about the need to formulate a diagnostic hypothesis immediately versus the need to allow time to obtain additional information.

As a consequence family physicians need recording methods and classification systems that cater to these specific needs and do not suffer from the problems formulated by White (1980, 1985) and at the same time reflect the state of the art in all branches of medicine.

## THE INTERNATIONAL CLASSIFICATION
## OF PRIMARY CARE

WONCA (World Organization of National Colleges, Academies and Academic Associations of General Practitioners/Family Physicians) provides an international forum to define the frame of reference of general practice and consequently to develop and field-test primary care classifications. ICHPPC-2 Defined, IC-Process-PC, and the International Glossary of Primary Care together form the basis of the International Classification of Primary Care (ICPC), which is WONCA's latest publication (Classification Committee of WONCA, 1981, 1983, 1986; Lamberts & Wood, 1987). ICPC is a system developed to classify simultaneously three of the four elements of the problem-oriented SOAP-registration:

1. *S* stands for the Subjective experience by patients of their problems, their demand for care, and their reason for encounter as this is clarified by the provider.
2. *O* stands for Objective findings—cannot be classified with ICPC.
3. *A* stands for Assessment or diagnostic interpretation of the patient's problem by the provider.
4. *P* stands for Process of care, representing the diagnostic and therapeutic interventions.

ICPC is the result of almost 10 years of development and field testing by an international group of taxonomers (most of them members of the Classification Committee of WONCA) with considerable experience in both primary and hospital care. The new classification incorporates a biaxial schema that permits the description and measurement of both the content and process of primary care in ambulatory and community settings (see Figure 4.1).

The integration of such data from numerous sources requires a degree of standardization of its elements in order to produce comparable, statistical information. This classification provides one such tool by incorporating the major rubrics and definitions of previously published classifications such as ICHPPC-2 Defined, the IC-Process-PC, and the draft WHO Reason for Encounter Classification (Classification Committee of WONCA, 1983, 1986; World Health Organization, 1981). It incorporates a manual for use in four modes (Reason for Encounter, Procedural, Diagnostic, and Comprehensive), a tabular list, a list of abbreviated titles, and an alphabetic index, which includes over 5,000 synonyms in English.

The simplicity of ICPC is based on its biaxial structure: 17 chapters in one axis, each with an alpha code; and seven identical components with rubrics bearing a two-digit numeric code, in the second axis.

The 17 chapters with their alpha codes are concerned with the following:

A  General and unspecific
B  Blood and blood-forming organs and lymphatics (spleen, bone marrow)
D  Digestive
E  Eye
H  Ear
K  Circulatory
L  Musculoskeletal
N  Neurological
P  Psychological
R  Respiratory
S  Skin
T  Endocrine, metabolic, and nutritional

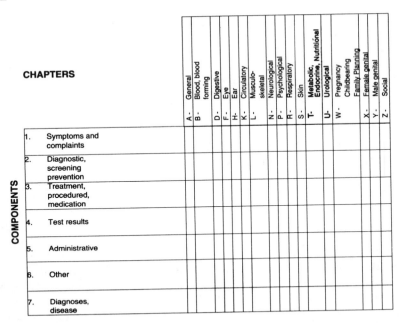

**Figure 4.1.** Biaxial Structure of ICPC: 17 Chapters and 7 Components

   U   Urological
   W   Pregnancy, child bearing, family planning
   X   Female genital (including breasts)
   Y   Male genital
   Z   Social

The seven components standard for each chapter are the following:

1. Complaint and symptom component
2. Diagnostic and preventive component
3. Treatment, procedures, and medication component
4. Test results component
5. Administrative component
6. Referral and other reasons for encounter component
7. Diagnosis and disease component, including:

   infectious disease
   neoplasms
   injuries
   congenital anomalies
   other specific diseases

ICPC has a significant mnemonic quality, particularly for components 2-6. This facilitates its day-to-day use both by physicians and other primary care providers and simplifies the centralized manual coding of data recorded elsewhere.

## The Development of ICPC as a Comprehensive Classification

Disease classifications are designed to allow the health care provider's interpretation of a patient's health problem to be coded in the form of an illness, disease, or injury. In contrast, a Reason for Encounter Classification focuses on data elements from the patient's perspective. In this respect it is patient-oriented rather than disease- or provider-oriented because the reasons for encounter (i.e., the demand for care) given by the patient have to be clarified by the physician or other health care worker before any attempt is made to interpret and assess the problem in terms of a diagnosis or to make any decision about the process of management and care (World Health Organization, 1984).

To begin this work, WHO called together a group of individuals experienced both in the provision of primary health care and in taxonomy. This group first met in Geneva in 1978. After 2 year's work they first produced the predecessor of ICPC, the Reason for Encounter Classification (RFEC), in field test form (World Health Organization, 1981).

The first field trial to test the completeness and reliability of the RFEC (now known as the Reason for Encounter Mode of ICPC) was a pilot study carried out in The Netherlands in 1980 (Lamberts, Meads, & Wood, 1984). The results obtained prompted further feasibility testing, which was carried out in nine countries: Australia, Brazil, Barbados, Hungary, Malaysia, The Netherlands, Norway, the United States, and the Philippines (Lamberts, Meads, & Wood, 1985). The developing world was well represented by Brazil, Barbados, Malaysia, and the Philippines, and recorders in all countries found the classification easy to use.

The entire classification was translated from English into several languages, including French, Hungarian, Norwegian, Portuguese, and Russian. The analysis of more than 90,000 reasons for encounter recorded during over 75,000 individual encounters, and the collective experience of the participants in eight countries (all except the Philippines), resulted in the development of a more comprehensive classification (Working Party on ICPC, 1985).

In the course of the feasibility testing, it was noted that RFEC could be used easily to classify simultaneously the reasons for encounter with two other elements of the problem-oriented care, namely the process and the assessment. Thus this conceptual framework allowed the evolution of the RFEC into the ICPC (Lamberts & Wood, 1987; Working Party on ICPC, 1985).

## Definitions

The basis for the use of ICPC as a diagnostic classification is the application of ICHPPC-2-Defined (Classification Committee of WONCA, 1983). Where a rubric is defined in ICHPPC-2, the same inclusion and exclusion criteria are to be used for ICPC. At present about two thirds of the rubrics in Component 7 have limited inclusion criteria available, which do not reach the level of specificity required for establishing a clinically absolute diagnosis, but do manifest those criteria that must invariably be present to allow use of that rubric. This manifestation enables measures of the "certainty" of the physician's use of these rubrics for diagnostic purposes. Terminological definition is an important new development in taxonomy and is an essential need for establishing more rigorous standards for research in primary care settings. Plans are to expand terminological definitions to the majority of rubrics in both Components 1 and 7 when they are used for diagnostic purposes.

Further, the coding rules of ICHPPC-2 are to be followed. The version of ICPC developed for relevance studies has been tested in the Transition Project carried out in The Netherlands since 1987, covering 12,750 patient years and approximately 34,000 encounters (Lamberts et al., 1987). Experiences from this project have been used—together with the results from the conversion study described below—to finalize ICPC in the form now published.

## ICPC as a Process Classification

The initial development work on a Reason for Encounter Classification focused on the patient-physician interaction during the encounter. Inevitably the need to identify administrative, investigative, and therapeutic interventions was required, which led to the formulation of Components 2-6, which structured the major elements of the process of care. Each rubric in these components was given a mnemonic quality, in that the two-digit numeric code was the same throughout all chapters. These major rubrics were similar to those incorporated in the IC-Process-PC.

# Optional Hierarchical Expansion

Clearly no single international classification can fulfill every need for every user; inevitably users sometimes will want to separate out certain problems contained in a single rubric. If this need arises, either because of increased incidence of a problem in one area or because of the special interests of the recorder, it can be solved by assigning special "in-house" code numbers to that problem and listing them under the original rubric.

This listing can be used for special studies over short periods of time or retained as a permanent expansion of the original rubric to meet special interests. A source for this expansion is usually a more detailed classification, such as the ICD-9 in the case of ICPC Components 1 and 7. For Components 2-6 the subrubrics available in IC-Process-PC can be used for expansion, as the major rubrics in both classifications are similar.

## THE RELATIONSHIP BETWEEN ICPC AND OTHER DIAGNOSTIC CLASSIFICATIONS

ICPC as a diagnostic classification system has relations both with ICD-9 and with other ICD-9-derived systems being used in primary care (Royal College of General Practitioners, 1984; World Health Organization, 1977). In order to understand the compatibility and comparability of ICPC with other systems, the codes of the rubrics in its first and seventh components (including their synonyms, as they can be found in the index) have been converted to the corresponding rubrics of three other diagnostic classification systems.

- the International Classification of Health Problems in Primary Care (ICHPPC-2). (An asterisk added to the ICHPPC position number indicates those ICHPPC-2 rubrics that are defined with the help of inclusion criteria (Classification Committee of WONCA, 1983).)
- the Classification of Diseases, Problems and Procedures, 1984, Royal College of General Practitioners (RCC) (Royal College of General Practitioners, 1984)
- the International Classification of Diseases, 9th Revision (ICD-9) (World Health Organization, 1977)

The conversion is only in one direction: from ICPC to the other systems. As a consequence only the conversion from ICPC to ICHPPC-2 covers all rubrics of the latter; the conversions to RCC and to ICD-9 cover most but not all rubrics of these two classification systems.

*Compatibility* is defined as "the capability of existing together in harmony; the ability to interrelate in an established consistent manner." *Comparability* is "the quality or state of being equivalent or similar." Compatibility was achieved and, to some extent, comparability, as will be demonstrated in the following paragraphs.

Several signs (plus, minus, or zero) indicate the degree of compatibility between the several codes. They are interpreted as follows:

- When a conversion is possible on a one-to-one basis and the corresponding rubric is similar, the systems are completely compatible for the rubric.
- A plus sign (+) indicates that the component of this rubric is less specific than that of the corresponding ICPC rubric; that is, the ICPC is more specific.
- A minus sign (−) indicates the reverse situation: The corresponding rubric is more specific than the ICPC rubric.
- When an ICPC rubric is incompatible with the other classification, this is indicated with a zero (0) or a plus-minus (+ −) sign. A "zero" rubric cannot be found in the other classifications. This lack does not necessarily mean, however, that conversion is absolutely impossible. All classifications have "grab bag" rubrics, which can absorb a variety of codes.
- A plus-minus (+ −) sign means that an ICPC rubric cannot be satisfactorily and logically converted to the other classification system because the relationship is too heterogeneous—both more and less specific elements simultaneously.

Attempted conversion of the first and seventh components of ICPC to the two primary care classifications, ICHPPC-2 and RCC, showed that ICPC as a diagnostic classification differed considerably from both. The rubrics of component 1 (322 symptoms and complaints) are relatively seldom replicated on a one-to-one basis: 14% in ICHPPC-2 or 16% in RCC. Many rubrics in component 1 are more specific than the corresponding rubrics in ICHPPC-2 (45%) or RCC (33%).

The 363 diagnostic rubrics in component 7 of ICPC correspond well with ICHPPC-2, as would be expected. In component 7, however, 48% of the ICPC rubrics are more specific than the corresponding ICHPPC-2 rubrics.

The specificity of the RCC in component 7 is slightly higher than that of ICPC, but different. The percentage of rubrics with a mixed compatibility is considerable (13%). The overall conclusion is that the compatibility and—because of the definitions—the comparability of ICPC with ICHPPC-2 are good.

Compared with ICHPPC-2, the distribution of the etiological diagnoses over the seventh component of the chapters of ICPC is responsible for most of its specificity. Etiological diagnoses in ICPC, however, can be lumped readily together to the corresponding ICHPPC-2 rubrics. The inclusion criteria of ICHPPC-2 Defined can be used in both systems, which makes their data highly comparable.

The RCC does not rely on inclusion criteria for the use of its rubrics, which diminishes its comparability with ICPC and ICHPPC-2. The comparability and compatibility of diagnostic information collected and analyzed with ICPC and RCC are also limited because of the relatively strong orientation of the latter to specific morphological diagnoses (Kay, 1984).

ICD-9 can still be recognized in the structure of ICPC and especially in its nomenclature. When patient-oriented information from primary care settings is collected and analyzed, however, ICPC and ICD-9 are practically compatible.

## Discussion

ICPC is a new system with a great potential for research and the structuring of patient-oriented clinical data. It describes the content of general practice/family medicine as it has developed over the years within the international view of WONCA. It is a relatively sophisticated tool and has been shown to work well in practice, but like all tools will not work equally well in every context (Lamberts et al., 1987). It works well in office practice settings and in any system involving such settings; therefore it is ideal for primary care practice networks, for the collection and management of clinical data in community settings, as the basic clinical classification for use in billing-linked systems reporting reimbursement data in terms of ICD-9, and for any context in which the patient has direct access to a primary care provider. It has been found useful in the analysis of health survey data culled from general populations, of clinical data collected from emergency room settings, and of encounter data on episodes of care.

An important conclusion is that the compatibility of the ICPC (and consequently also of the defined rubrics of the ICHPPC-2) with the RCC (and therefore even more so with the ICD-9) is limited. The number of main rubrics that can be converted directly is rather small; also, the direction of specificity means that for many rubrics only an incomplete conversion is possible (+ −sign). Once a particular classification system is selected, the capacity to compare results with those from another system is at best limited.

Another important conclusion is the abandoning of the idea that a technical solution to the problem of limited compatibility can be found through the use of a computerized nomenclature with the various conversion codes. It may be useful, however, to establish a generally accepted and widely applicable computer thesaurus based on a nomenclature structure of each of the classification systems discussed here. To initiate this development, Oxford University Press has arranged to publish a diskette along with the Manual for Use of ICPC that covers the relevant conversions possible with ICPC.

An important question will be whether WONCA will decide to further develop its classification needs along the lines of ICPC, which as a consequence will lead to less compatibility with the concept of ICD (Anonymous, 1984; World Health Organization, 1984). The proposed structure of ICD-10 poses even more problems for primary care physicians than does its predecessor (World Health Organization, 1986).

Therefore the editors of ICPC propose to develop a strategy for integrating ICD-10 and a second version of ICPC in terms of their comparability and compatibility at the levels of terminology, nomenclature classification, and a technical conversion at the thesaurus level for computer systems, as was done with ICD-9. These various levels will be illustrated by examples.

Such a system should enable the collection of episode-oriented data from different primary care settings in many countries, which when classified with ICPC, will improve documentation and decision making (Classification Committee of WONCA, 1983; White, 1985).

## References

Anonymous. (1984). New classification of diseases and problems. *Journal of Collective General Practice, 34,* 125-127.

Classification Committee of WONCA. (1981). An international glossary for primary care. *Journal of Family Practice, 13,* 671-681.

Classification Committee of WONCA. (1983). *ICHPPC-2 Defined: Inclusion criteria for the use of the rubrics of the international classification of health problems in primary care.* Oxford, UK: Oxford University Press.

Classification Committee of WONCA. (1986). *International classification of process in primary care IC-Process-PC.* Oxford, UK: Oxford University Press.

Green, L. A., Wood, M., Becker, L., Farley, E. S., Jr., Freeman, W. L., Froom, J., Hames, C., Niebauer, L. J., Rosser, W. W., & Seifert, M. (1984). The ambulatory sentinal practice network: Purpose, methods and policies. *Journal of Family Practice, 18,* 275-280.

Kay, C. R. (1984). RCGP Classification. *Family Practice, 3,* 66-67.

Kilpatrick, S. J., & Boyle, R. M. (Eds.). (1984). *Primary care research: Encounter records and the denominator problem.* New York: Praeger.

Lamberts, H. (1984). *Morbidity in general practice: Diagnosis-related information from the monitoring project.* Utrecht, Netherlands: Huisartsenpers bv.

Lamberts, H., Brouwer, H. J., Groen, A. S. M., & Huisman, H. (1987). Het Transitiemodel in de Huisartspraktijk. Praktisch Gebruik van de ICPC Tijdens 28,000 Contacten. *Huisarts en Wetenschap, 30,* 105-113.

Lamberts, H., Meads, S., & Wood, M. (1984). Classification of reasons why persons seek primary care: Pilot study of a new system. *Public Health Report, 99,* 587-597.

Lamberts, H., Meads, S., & Wood, M. (1985). Results of the international field trial with the reason for encounter classification. *Sozial-und Praventivmedizin, 30,* 80-87.

Lamberts, H., & Schade, E. (1988). Surveillance systems from primary care data: From a prevalence-oriented epidemiology. In W. J. Eylenbosch & N. D. Noah (Eds.), *Surveillance in health disease.* Oxford, UK: Oxford University Press.

Lamberts, H., & Wood, M. (Eds.). (1987). *International classification of primary care.* Oxford: Oxford University Press.

National Center for Health Services and Health Care Technology Assessment. (1985). *Program for Health Services Research on Primary Care.* Atlanta, GA: U.S. Department of Health and Human Services.

Royal College of General Practitioners. (1975). *Morbidity statistics for general practice.* London: Royal College of General Practitioners, Office of Population Censuses and Surveys.

Royal College of General Practitioners. (1984). *Classification of diseases, problems and procedures 1984* (Occasional Paper 26). London: Royal College of General Practitioners.

White, K. L. (1980). Information for health care: An epidemiological perspective. *Inquiry, 17,* 296-312.

White, K. L. (1985). Restructuring the international classification of diseases: Need for a new paradigm. *Journal of Family Practice, 21,* 17-20.

Working Party on ICPC. (1985). *International classification of primary care (ICPC): Manual for use of ICPC in relevance studies.* Amsterdam: University of Amsterdam, Department of General Practice.

Working Party on RFEC. (1981). *Report to develop a classification of the "Reason for contact with primary health care services."* Geneva: World Health Organization.

World Health Organization. (1977). *International classification of diseases (9th rev.).* Geneva: Author.

World Health Organization. (1984). *International conference of health statistics for the year 2000: Report of WHO on a Bellagio Conference.* Budapest: WHO Statistical Publishing House.

World Health Organization. (1986). *ICD-10-proposal.* Geneva: Author.

# 5 Selecting an Instrument to Measure the Outcomes of Health Care

DAVID WILKIN

## Introduction

The emphasis placed over the past decade or so on controlling health care costs has created a powerful stimulus for research into the effectiveness and efficiency of health services. This in turn has generated a wide range of measures designed in varying degrees to estimate the needs for and the outcomes of health care. The practitioner or researcher who is concerned with selecting an appropriate instrument for a particular purpose is faced with an Aladdin's cave of measures covering most aspects of the consequences of disease, but the right choice has to be made. A number of excellent reviews of instruments have been written (Hersen & Bellack, 1988; Kane & Kane, 1981; McDowell & Newell, 1987; Teeling Smith, 1988; Walker & Rosser, 1988). The main purpose of this chapter, however, is to offer intending users some guidance about the criteria that should be applied when considering which instruments will best meet their needs. And, since the selection of an instrument is only one of the tasks of measuring outcomes of medical care, it is important first to devote some attention to the concept of outcome and to the key elements in conducting research into outcomes.

The dictionary definition of *outcome* is simply "result or visible effect." To be concerned with outcomes is simply to be concerned with the causal relationships between antecedent and subsequent conditions or events. But in the context of health and illness, outcome is usually defined in terms of the achievement of, or failure to achieve, desired goals. In order to demonstrate the existence of a relationship between the provision of medical care and these desired goals, a number of important issues must be addressed.

## DESCRIBING THE NATURAL HISTORY

Whatever the problem under study (commonly although not always defined in terms of disease categories), it should be possible to describe its natural history; that is, the course it would take without health care intervention. This natural history provides a baseline against which outcomes can be measured. For example, it is possible to measure the effectiveness of health care for acute appendicitis in terms of case fatality, since the natural history of untreated appendicitis is known. If no effective treatment is known, such as for the common cold, it is difficult to see how the effectiveness of a new treatment could be evaluated without reference to its natural history. Unfortunately it is rare that such information is available in a systematic form.

An alternative to plotting the natural history is to use as a baseline the history of the condition under existing patterns of care. For example, the efficacy of new drugs usually is assessed against the standard that is set by drugs already available, rather than in terms of the natural history of the condition without treatment.

## DEFINING THE OBJECTIVES
## OF HEALTH CARE

At the most general level, the objective of health care could be said to be the improvement of health or a reduction in the level of ill health. This objective is not very helpful, however, when it comes to attempts to evaluate the effectiveness of specific interventions. Objectives can be stated at different levels of aggregation, from the individual to the family to the community to society as a whole. They may refer to different time periods (the present, the immediate future, a lifetime), and they will reflect the differing values of interested parties. In some instances a clear and overriding immediate objective will be agreed to by all parties (e.g., to keep the patient alive following a heart attack), but such instances are rare, and often agreement is only transitory. Explicitly defined objectives are much less common in primary medical care than in many other specialties. For most problems a wide range of possible objectives exists that will be awarded different values and priorities by different interested parties (patient, doctor, nurse, relatives, friends, etc.). When launching research to look at outcomes, it is important to ask *who* is defining the objectives that determine the selection of outcome criteria. If this question is not asked, a danger exists that the measures selected will reflect primarily the objectives of professionals. For example, many studies of cancer treatments have focused solely on survival rates, regardless of the quality of life experienced by patients and their relatives.

## DESCRIBING INPUTS

There is little point in attempting to measure outcomes without being able to provide a precise description of inputs, since the term *outcome* implies the existence of a causal model that relates certain structures and/or processes to end results. Even apparently straightforward descriptions, such as whether a drug was prescribed, can become complicated. Was the drug subsequently dispensed, and if it was dispensed, did the patient take it as advised? When one is attempting to describe such inputs as diagnosis, counseling, reassurance, monitoring, and so on, the problems become infinitely more complex. Indeed, finding appropriate methods of measuring inputs can be more difficult than identifying suitable outcome measures. In most instances the attempt to measure inputs ends with a description of a relatively small range of service inputs. But inputs from other agencies and from informal sources can be at least as important.

## SPECIFYING THE RELATIONSHIP
## BETWEEN INPUTS AND OUTCOMES

Although it is possible to examine the relationship between inputs and outcomes without clearly specifying the nature of that relationship, doing so is likely to leave important questions unanswered. For example, evidence might be produced to support the hypothesis that routine follow-up of patients suffering from asthma results in fewer symptoms. While such a finding might be useful, it is difficult to interpret. Does follow-up achieve better outcomes because the medication is reviewed and modified as appropriate, or because patient compliance is improved? If it is compliance that is important, is this importance a function of increased knowledge, or a fear of being reprimanded? In either case it may be that follow-up is not the best method of achieving the desired outcome. Research into the outcomes of health care will be of much greater value if it can go beyond the crude demonstration of statistical associations between particular patterns of care and outcomes. In order to do this, it is necessary to devote more attention at the planning stage to the clear formulation of questions or hypotheses that attempt to specify the intermediate steps between inputs and outcomes, in ways that make it possible to identify the strengths and weaknesses of the causal model.

## RESEARCH DESIGN

Since it is impossible to measure accurately, or even be aware of, all potentially confounding variables when examining the relationship between the provision of health care and the outcomes of that care, the selection of an appropriate research design is an important way of minimizing their effects. Unfortunately the use of the classic double-blind randomized controlled trial as a research design is only rarely possible in a complex system of health care. Many studies will be concerned with multidimensional problems and complex patterns, and in such circumstances it will be necessary to use either nonrandomized trials or observational studies. The two principal analytical approaches are comparisons of populations exposed and not exposed to defined patterns of care (prospective cohort studies), and those with and without the desired outcome (retrospective case control studies). The choice of research design will depend on many factors peculiar to the particular problem. The value of the work done to set objectives, to select appropriate outcome measures, to measure inputs, and so on, will be fully realized only if these are employed in an appropriate design.

## Criteria for Selection

In making a choice of measure, it is essential to have an understanding of the principles of measurement and thus to know what to look for in terms of the development and testing of an instrument. Measurement consists of the application of a set of rules for assigning values (usually numeric) to objects or events so as to represent quantities, qualities, or categories of attributes. The fact that rules are explicit and unambiguous implies an ability to standardize so that the same results will be obtained by different people using the same instrument. Moreover it is clearly essential that the instrument should actually measure what it is intended to measure. While these conditions may be unproblematic for many everyday measurements in the physical world, this is far from being the case for events and objects in the social world.

PURPOSE FOR WHICH MEASURE
IS REQUIRED

The purposes of health-related measures can be divided into three broad categories: discrimination, prediction, and evaluation (McDowell & Newell, 1987). Often a particular study may have more than one purpose, but it will be helpful when making a selection to distinguish between them.

Discrimination between individuals or groups on some underlying health-related dimension is commonly required, both as a means of describing differences in health experience and as a means of identifying areas of need. For example, if one wants to know whether people in different social classes have different levels of health, one requires a measure that is capable of detecting differences between groups. More practically, a policy of selective allocation of resources will require data collected using a discriminative index in order to be able to target those groups or areas where needs are greatest.

Measures are commonly employed in medicine as a means of identifying groups or individuals who have or will develop some target condition or outcome. That is, they are used to predict future needs. Screening tests such as cervical smears or developmental tests for children are used to identify problems at an earlier stage than they would otherwise manifest themselves. Other predictive measures are used because they are less uncomfortable or less costly than alternatives. Thus, for example, simple functional assessments may be used as indicators of needs for services by elderly people in the community. They are predictive both of more detailed assessments by health and social care professionals, and of successful outcomes, such as continued independent living.

The attention of researchers, practitioners, and policymakers increasingly has turned to the use of measures for purposes of evaluation. The evaluator requires a measure of the magnitude of longitudinal change on the dimension of interest. Whether the measure discriminates between individuals or groups or is able to predict future outcomes is not important. Attention is focused on changes between point A and point B that are attributable to particular interventions: outcomes. This focus is the purpose of clinical trials and of more broadly based service evaluations. Survival rates and cure rates are classic measures of medical outcome for evaluative research, but many measures of health and quality of life can also be used.

Within these broad categories of purpose are a variety of subcategories that also can have a bearing on measurement criteria. The most important of these criteria are whether one is concerned with individuals or groups, and the magnitude of the differences/outcomes that are the focus of interest. The clinician or practitioner is primarily concerned with individuals and thus will require measures capable of detecting differences at this level. The researcher, on the other hand, often requires a lower level of precision, being interested in group differences. A less precise measure will be required to detect a real difference between two groups of 100 people than between two individuals. But the level of precision required will be determined also by the expected magnitude of differences.

## LEVEL OF MEASUREMENT

Four distinct levels of measurement exist: nominal, ordinal, interval, and ratio. The interpretations that can be placed on results and the ways in which they can be manipulated in analyses are dependent on the level of measurement achieved. It is essential therefore to choose an instrument that achieves a level of measurement that will permit the sorts of analyses required of it.

*Nominal scales* represent the categorical level of measurement. They consist of systematic identification and labeling of classes of objects or events. At one extreme the classification male/female is a nominal scale for sex; at the other the International Classification of Diseases (ICD) is a nominal scale for classifying all diagnoses and presenting problems. The fact that numbers may be attached to different values for practical purposes (e.g., 1 male, 2 female) does not imply any ordering or other inherent relationship between values. That is, it would be equally valid to code females=1 and males=2 or to reverse the numeric codes employed in the ICD. Nominal scales can be used only to determine *how often* an event or attribute occurs.

*Ordinal scales* differ from nominal in that their descriptions of classes of objects or events are ordered along a continuum of some sort (e.g., least to most, worst to best). An ordinal scale does not permit the user to determine how far apart are points on the scale but simply to hierarchically rank each point. Perhaps the most common sort of ordinal scale in medicine is "severe, moderate, mild" as a means of classifying the severity of disease. We know that moderate is worse than mild and severe is worse than moderate, but we do not know by how much. Neither do we know how far they are from absolute values at either end of the spectrum. Thus knowing that a person suffers from "mild" arthritis tells us nothing about how far away that person is from complete health at one end of the spectrum or death at the other. Scores on ordinal scales cannot be added or subtracted, and it is therefore not appropriate to apply even basic statistics such as means or standard deviations unless scaling techniques have been used to convert them to higher order scales. It would be meaningless, for example, to rate arthritic patients on a one-to-three scale (mild to severe) and calculate an average for a group of patients.

*Interval scales* not only provide a rank ordering but also specify the distance between points on the scale. They do not, however, provide an absolute zero point. Temperature measured in Fahrenheit or Celsius is a good example of an interval scale. It is possible to add or subtract values and thus calculate basic statistics, such as the average daytime temperature in Manchester, but the absence of an absolute zero means that scores on an interval scale cannot be multiplied or divided. Thus it is incorrect to say that a temperature of 60 is twice as hot as a temperature of 30. Many measures of health-related variables claim to be at the interval level, but such claims are often open to question.

*Ratio scale* is the fourth level of measurement. In addition to meeting all the criteria for an interval scale, it has an absolute zero point or defined point of origin. This point permits values to be multiplied or divided. Time and distance measures are examples of ratio scales. Not only is it possible to calculate the mean age of a group, it is also legitimate to say that a person of 60 years is twice as old as someone of 30 years.

Recognition of the differences between levels of measurement is important because of their respective limitations. The level of measurement achieved will determine the appropriate level of analysis. It is, unfortunately, all too common to see results of ordinal or even nominal levels of measurement subjected to wholly inappropriate statistical analyses.

## TYPE OF MEASURE AND CONSTRUCTION

To understand the strengths and limitations of a measure, including the level of measurement achieved, it helps to know how it was constructed. All the measures included in subsequent chapters consist of a number of questions or items, responses to which are scored and may be aggregated in some way to form either a single index or a number of values representing different dimensions. It is beyond the scope of this book to provide a detailed account of methods of constructing and testing scales, but the potential user should have at least a basic understanding of the terms commonly used.

*Single Item Versus Multi-item Measures.* The simplest measures employ a single item to measure a particular concept. This item may be as broad as, "How would you describe your health at present?" or as narrow as "How far are you able to walk without assistance?" Most instruments, however, are multi-item measures. They use a number of questions or statements, and responses are combined in some way to produce a score. Thus, for example, mobility might be covered by five items: walking, running, transfer from bed or chair, climbing stairs, and using public transport.

*Response Categories.* Whether a single item or a number of items is used, appropriate response categories must be provided. Response categories are of four basic types. First, questions can be phrased to produce simple yes/no responses. Second, a number of descriptions can be placed in rank order (e.g., unable to walk, walks less than 50 yards, can walk more than 50 yards). Third, responses to statements can be classified as a number of points on a single dimension (e.g., strongly agree, agree, neutral, disagree, strongly disagree). This type of response category is used in Likert scaling. The fourth method, the visual analog, is closely related. Here the respondent is presented with a line anchored at both ends and asked to place a mark anywhere on the line (e.g., *very sad*—————————*very happy*).

*Indexes versus Profiles.* The purpose of multi-item measures is to combine the items in some way in order to create a score or scores. In some cases all items relate to a single dimension and are therefore combined to produce a single score (e.g., depression). When a number of different dimensions are covered (e.g., mobility, household tasks, pain, emotional state), these can be either presented as separate scores (a profile) or combined to produce an aggregate score (an index). An index is an attempt to create a truly multidimensional measure. Some indexes are constructed so that scores can be presented either as profiles or as an overall score.

*Scaling Techniques.* A wide variety of scaling techniques has been used to construct measures of health status and patient satisfaction (e.g., rank ordering, Guttman scaling, Likert scaling, category rating or equal-appearing intervals, paired comparisons, utility estimation and magnitude estimation). Some, such as rank ordering and category rating, are closely related and might more properly be considered subdivisions of the same general approach. The choice of technique will depend on various considerations, such as whether the measure is unidimensional or multidimensional, the intended uses, the level of measurement required, theoretical considerations, and practical constraints in both development and use of the measure. It should be remembered that the method used will have been determined by the criteria applied by the original authors, which may not be the same as those of another researcher or practitioner seeking an "off the rack" instrument.

Scaling techniques are employed with varying degrees of rigor. In some cases development and testing bear only a passing resemblance to systematic techniques, and in others it appears an attempt has been made to use a formal psychometric approach.

*Item Generation.* The initial step with all measures based on self-report or descriptions of health states is to generate the questions, statements, or descriptions to be included in the instrument. Methods of doing this generation can be divided broadly into those that rely on professional judgments and those that draw directly or indirectly on the experiences of the people for whom the measure is intended, although in many instances elements of both are at work. It is surprising how many measures seem, at least in the first instance, to have been constructed solely on the basis of the authors' own experience. Somewhat more sophisticated are those that generate statements from a panel of professional judges or from the professional literature. In some instances this will be the most appropriate method. When the purpose is to measure subjective experience of needs or outcomes, however, the most appropriate technique is to ask intended respondents what problems they have experienced, how they rate these in terms of importance or severity, and what they feel are important criteria of need or outcome. This questioning can be done through semistructured interviews or group discussions or, more economically, by reviewing other studies that have reported the perceptions of target populations.

*Selection of Judges.* Many scaling methods require the use of judges both to select items and to allocate weights or values to items or states. Since the judgments of the judges will be fundamental to the validity of the scale, it is essential that these individuals be chosen carefully and that they are described adequately by the authors. Nonprofessional judges should be drawn from the population on whom the measure will be used. Other users should note that procedures for standardization and weighting derived from one group of judges may not be applicable in a different context (for example, weights derived from American judges may not apply in Britain). Also it should be noted that more sophisticated measurement procedures impose more complex tasks on the judges. It seems unlikely, for example, that utility estimation techniques such as the standard gamble could be applied in a general population sample.

*Item Reduction.* With scales derived from a large pool of items (whether generated by potential respondents or from existing literature), it will be necessary to reduce the number of items to manageable proportions. The standard scaling techniques described earlier are accompanied by standard techniques for item reduction based on consistency and representativeness. Thus, for example, in the analysis of initial versions of a Likert-type scale, those items that produce inconsistent responses are excluded. Statistical techniques often are employed to achieve item reduction. Procedures designed to measure internal consistency (see section on reliability, below) can be used to maximize the precision of an instrument to measure a given construct, and to reduce the number of items to a minimum. Such procedures are entirely appropriate for a measure designed to discriminate between groups. When a measure is required for evaluative purposes, however, the criteria for item reduction may be different. Measures of internal consistency focus on consistency *between* respondents at a point in time, but the evaluator is interested in consistency *within* individuals over a period of time. Also, for evaluative research it may be less important to minimize the number of items, and more important to ensure that any item that may show a difference is retained.

*Weighting.* Techniques for attributing weights to individual items in order to construct a total score are provided within each of the scaling methods. The purpose of differentially weighting items is to permit the inclusion of items at different levels of severity without distorting the overall scale score. Weights will be based on the importance attached to items by the judges, whatever the particular method of scaling used. It should be remembered that a different group of judges might produce different weights.

*Reliability.* One of the objectives of any measurement should be to reduce to a minimum both random and nonrandom error. All measurement includes some degree of random error (i.e., error that follows no systematic pattern). The more reliable a measure is, the lower the element of random error.

The reliability of a measure is the extent to which it yields the same results in repeated applications on an unchanged population or phenomenon. A speedometer that one day gives a reading of 70 mph, the next day 60 mph, and the third day 80 mph, although on all three occasions the car was traveling at 70 mph (the maximum speed limit on British roads) is clearly unreliable and therefore likely to expose the driver to the risk of a fine for speeding. The reliability of clinical, social, and psychological instruments is less easily established but equally or even more important. Three types of reliability are generally considered important in the assessment of instruments. First, consistency over time is assessed by using repeated applications of the instrument (test-retest reliability). Second, consistency between different users of the instrument may need to be established (interrater reliability). Third, the internal consistency of items within the instrument can be assessed (i.e., to what extent do all of the items measure the same dimension?). These are discussed in more detail by Ferris and Norton in Chapter 6.

## VALIDITY

The validity of an instrument relates to the effects of nonrandom or systematic error. Reliability is a necessary but not sufficient condition for a useful measure: a speedometer may be perfectly reliable if it always shows 70 mph when the true speed is 80 mph, but as the driver will find, when stopped by the police, it is not a valid indicator of the speed traveled. An instrument is valid to the extent that it measures what it purports to measure. Like reliability, validity is not determined in the abstract. A measure may be valid for the specific purpose for which it was developed, but not for a related purpose. The potential user of a measure should examine evidence of validity in the context of the practical use to which it is intended to put the measure. Validity is of three basic types: content, criterion, and construct. (See Ferris & Norton, Chapter 6, for a more detailed discussion of types of validity.)

## RESPONSIVENESS

In a series of papers concerning the usefulness of health status and quality-of-life measures as evaluative instruments, Guyatt and his colleagues (Guyatt, Bombardier, & Tugwell, 1986; Guyatt, Walters, & Norman, 1985; Kirshner & Guyatt, 1985) and Deyo (Deyo, 1984; Deyo & Inui, 1984) have drawn attention to the failure of existing measures to identify small but clinically significant changes. They have argued that the criteria for selecting a measure for evaluative purposes should include its sensitivity to change. Sensitivity or responsiveness is closely related to validity, and some authors include it under the heading of discriminant validity. Responsiveness, however, is not essential to validity; rather, it is a characteristic of the measure and is thus perhaps better dealt with separately.

Although responsiveness to clinically significant change in individuals over time is likely to be a major consideration in any study concerned with evaluating the impact of treatment, it tends not to be routinely included in the development of measures. Because the development of many measures of health and health related-variables has emphasized validity and reliability rather than responsiveness, information is often inadequate about how useful such measures would be in evaluative research. Indeed, the preferred methods of establishing validity and reliability tend to militate against responsiveness. They tend to focus on the ability to discriminate between individuals or groups, on correlation with other measures, and on internal consistency. Measures that are good at discriminating tend to have very limited response categories (e.g., yes/no) to minimize the problem of respondents placing different interpretations on response categories. They tend to exclude items that only apply to small numbers of respondents, and they keep the number of items to a minimum in order to maximize internal consistency. In contrast, a measure that is responsive to small changes over time in the same individuals may require a more refined grading of responses to items and the inclusion of any item that might show change. Such a measure may be poor at discriminating between groups; it may exclude items that are good discriminators but not amenable to change; and it may include others that only affect a few respondents or are treated inconsistently. Nevertheless, it may be perfectly valid as a measure of change in individuals.

## ADMINISTRATION AND PRACTICAL ISSUES

While scientific criteria are vitally important in the selection of an appropriate measure, they should not be applied to the exclusion of more practical considerations. The choice of the best measure for a particular job will often be a compromise between scientific rigor and practical constraints. Researchers need to consider the practical problems of administering the measure, both from their own point of view, from the point of view of the respondents, and in relation to problems of analyzing data once these have been collected.

Perhaps the most important decision is whether the measure is to be self-administered by respondents or administered by an interviewer. Clearly the time savings are considerable for the researcher if his or her presence is not required; the measures can be distributed by mail or given to respondents in the course of other activities (e.g., consultation, clinic attendance). In contrast, the interviewer-administered measure by definition requires either the researcher or a qualified interviewer to be present, and the constraints of time and resources inevitably mean that a far smaller number of responses will be obtained than with a postal questionnaire. It is likely also that the study would have to be restricted to a small geographical area. Against these considerations are undoubted advantages to interviewer-administered measures. First, although the total number of respondents will be smaller, the response rate (the proportion of those approached who actually respond) will be higher. Second, it will be possible to collect more information from each respondent, perhaps using a variety of measures and some open-ended questions. Third, it is possible in a face-to-face interview to deal with sensitive issues that would be difficult or impossible to raise through the impersonal medium of a mailed questionnaire. The choice between these two methods will depend on the particular objectives and circumstances of the study.

Related to the problem of method of administration is the issue of proxy responses. If the research deals with severely ill or infirm people, instances will arise in which the intended respondent is unable to complete the measure or unwilling to be interviewed. Rather than treating such cases as nonrespondents, the researcher may wish to complete the measures using information from a third party (e.g., spouse, other relative, nurse, or residential care worker). Indeed it is not uncommon, even when the respondent is able to answer the questions, to find that a relative or friend "helps" with the answers. Some measures are intended to be completed by a third party and thus present no problem, but most are intended to be completed by the respondent, and evidence of their reliability and validity is based on their being applied in this way. Thus if third-party responses are to be used, they should be clearly identified for analysis. If third- party responses are likely to be a common problem, it may be worth mounting a study to test the use of the measure in this way.

Whatever the measure chosen and the method of administration, it is essential to calculate carefully the resources required for administration. These resources will include the time taken to draw a sample, negotiating access with appropriate authorities, printing and stationery costs, postage, traveling time, and costs of following up nonrespondents. Even the most experienced researchers tend to underestimate how much time and effort is necessary for the successful administration of a survey questionnaire. It is always advisable, however small the study, to carry out a small pretest in order to calculate exactly how much time has to be allocated for each task. In calculating the resources required, the researcher should not forget the demands being made on respondents and others. Respondents will be asked to devote some of their time and energy to helping the researcher, usually free of charge. Is it reasonable to expect them to give up their time, particularly if they are feeling unwell? If the demands are unreasonable, it is likely that a substantial proportion will refuse to complete the measure. For example, asking patients to complete a lengthy questionnaire immediately after a visit to the doctor is unlikely to generate a high response rate.

One of the most commonly ignored issues at the planning stage of research is how the data will be processed and analyzed. The golden rule should be to avoid collecting data that will not be used, either because of the quantity collected or the complexity of analysis required. In selecting a measure, the researcher should consider carefully how the information is to be processed and how it will be used in analyses. Even the basic entry of data into a computer can be extremely time-consuming for a large-scale study. Although most of the measures reviewed in later chapters provide for relatively straightforward analysis, it is likely that they will form only part of a larger battery of questions and tests. In these circumstances the researcher should have a clear idea at the outset of how the information can be used so that any redundant items can be excluded at this stage.

## Conclusion

No measure will perform well against all the criteria discussed in this chapter: they all have strengths and weaknesses that make them more or less suitable for particular purposes. The prospective user of measures of outcomes in the field of health care does not need to become an expert in the various aspects of research methodology discussed here. A knowledge of the basic principles involved in the design and testing of measures is required, however, in order to be able to make an informed choice and to use the chosen measure appropriately.

## References

Deyo, R. A. (1984). Measuring functional outcomes in therapeutic trials for chronic disease. *Controlled Clinical Trials, 5,* 223-240.

Deyo, R. A., & Inui, T. S. (1984). Toward clinical applications of health status measures: Sensitivity of scales to clinically important changes. *Health Services Research, 19*(3), 277-289.

Guyatt, G., Bombardier, C., & Tugwell, P. (1986). Measuring disease specific quality of life in clinical trials. *Canadian Medical Association Journal, 134,* 889-895.

Guyatt, G., Walters, S., & Norman, G. (1985). Measuring change over time: Assessing the usefulness of evaluative instruments. *Journal of Chronic Diseases, 40*(2), 171-178.

Hersen, M. & Bellack, A. S. (Eds.). (1988). *Dictionary of behavioural assessment techniques.* New York: Pergamon.

Kane, R. A., & Kane, R. L. (1981). *Assessing the elderly: A practical guide to measurement.* Lexington, MA: Lexington.

Kirshner, B., & Guyatt, G. (1985). A methodological framework for assessing health indices. *Journal of Chronic Diseases, 38,* 27-36.

McDowell, I., & Newell, C. (1987). *Measuring health: A guide to rating scales and questionnaires.* New York: Oxford University Press.

Teeling Smith, G. (Ed.). (1988). *Measuring health: A practical approach.* Chichester, UK: John Wiley.

Walker, S. R., & Rosser, R. M. (Eds.). (1988). *Quality of life: Assessment and application.* Lancaster, UK: MPT Press.

# 6  Basic Concepts in Reliability and Validity

LORRAINE E. FERRIS
PETER G. NORTON

## Introduction

Standardized questionaires are used in the health care field to assist in making decisions about selection, classification, and evaluation of educational or treatment procedures. Primary care researchers commonly use such questionnaires to select individuals who meet some inclusion criterion, to classify patients for the purpose of placement or diagnosis, and to evaluate treatments or outcomes of intervention.

A standardized test is one in which the procedure, apparatus, scoring, norms, and reliability and validity properties have been established and confirmed through empirical investigation. When planning a research project, the investigator may be required to evaluate a number of potential tests and to select the one that is most appropriate. Any of the above dimensions may preclude or favor the use of a particular test, but the strength of the last two is particularly important. It is through evaluation of reliability and validity—the psychometric properties that researchers use to decide on the number and kind of conclusions they are prepared to make based on their data. (Note that some researchers opt for terminology other than *psychometrics* to connote the establishment of reliability and validity properties.) Using tests with sound psychometric properties also makes comparisons between different studies more legitimate and helps researchers build on previous knowledge.

This chapter presents an overview of psychometrics in an effort to sensitize novice researchers to the conceptual underpinnings. Since the area is both conceptually and statistically complex, the discussion will focus only on basic concepts; expert consultation should be sought when planning a research endeavor and, if warranted, throughout the study. As additional resources, readers are advised to consult the chapters in this volume by Zyzanski (Chapter 9) and by Tudiver and Ferris (Chapter 8).

## What Is Psychometrics?

Psychometrics refers to those statistical methods that empirically investigate whether a test measures what is intended (validity) and yields consistent findings over time (reliability). These methods produce quantitative indices that represent both the amount and type of reliability and validity associated with a test. The field originated in psychology, and new psychometric techniques are continually being developed and refined by psychologists. These techniques have been extended to other fields, however, and have been used to verify instruments that measure symptoms, physical signs, and patient-related variables: in fact, many if not most of the input and outcome variables in primary care. (A particular focus has been to attempt to measure psychological attributes as they relate to physical health.) The issues of what is being measured in these indices, how well it is being measured, and the consistency in results over time are of great importance.

## Basic Concepts in Psychometrics

*Reliability* measures assess the range of fluctuation likely to occur in an individual's score as a result of chance errors; that is, the repeatability of results. This chapter will examine five types of reliability: coefficient alpha, split-half technique, test-retest, alternative forms, and interrater and examiner reliability. The *validity* of a test refers to what the test measures and how well it measures it. Four types of validity are considered here: content validity, face validity, criterion-related validity (concurrent or predictive), and construct validity.

Two types of measurement errors can affect reliability and validity. Reliability is affected by *random errors*, which temporarily produce a bias in the measure due to transient changes in the respondent, situation, or methodology. Validity is affected both by random error and by *systematic* or *constant error*, which biases a measure in a particular direction and thereby affects the construct being measured or the measurement process. An example is when respondents have a particular "response set" —perhaps always answering yes-no questions with a no, or always answering Likert questions (scored on a 1-to-5-point scale) with one of the extreme values or the middle point, or zigzagging across response options without regard to the content. These types of content-free response sets are referred to as *acquiescent response sets*. Another type of constant error results from a respondent's attempts to answer a questionnaire in a way that is socially desirable or believed to be the preferred answer. This is referred to as *social desirability*. A valid instrument minimizes the amount of systematic error by ensuring that it measures the underlying structure of the concepts of interest.

## Reliability

Measures of test reliability estimate the proportion of the total variance of test results that is attributable to true differences in the phenomenon under consideration, and not to *error variance*. What is a true difference and what is due to error is contingent on the construct under consideration and the purpose of the test: *Error variance* is defined as "any condition that is deemed to be irrelevant." This definition emphasizes the importance of reducing error variance by controlling for any factors that may create "noise" in the measurement; for example, having standard testing conditions for the setting, instructions, and time limits. A familiar example is the care with which blood pressure must be measured. Using a random zero sphygmomanometer, having the patient rest in supine position for 5 minutes prior to measurement, and taking the average of three consecutive readings will produce a reliable measure. Clearly, however, in a clinical setting this kind of control is usually impossible. Similar problems are encountered in applying paper-and-pencil tests, semistructured interviews, and in fact in almost any measure used in research. Even in the ideal world it is not possible to control for all sources of error variance. It is for this reason that the calculation and interpretation of a reliability index are essential.

Reliability is expressed as a coefficient that ranges from 0 to 1: The larger the error variance, the smaller the coefficient. Thus it is equal to 1 if no measurement error occurs, and 0 if all the variance in a score is due to error. Unlike other types of coefficients that have to be squared in order to represent the amount of variance explained, reliability coefficients are directly interpreted: For example, a reliability coefficient of .80 signifies that 80% of the variance depends on true variance, while 20% depends on error variance.

The different types of reliability differ in the sources of error variance identified. Briefly, *coefficient alpha* is expressed by a reliability coefficient that reflects the estimate of the split-half correlation for all possible combinations of dividing the test. The *split-half technique for internal consistency* yields a coefficient that represents a correlation between the scores on an arbitrary half of the measure, with the scores on the other half. In recent years psychometric experts usually only employ split-half reliability when items are scored dichotomously (Nunnally, 1978). It is rarely used even when items are categorical, because different results can be obtained depending on how the test is halved. The *test-retest for stability* correlates the scores obtained on repeated administrations of the test. *Alternate* or *parallel forms* yield a correlation coefficient between scores on two equivalent forms administered in immediate succession. Finally, *interrater reliability* refers to the consistency of ratings of the same individual by different raters.

## COEFFICIENTS OF CONSISTENCY: SPLIT-HALF AND COEFFICIENT ALPHA RELIABILITY

Internal-consistency coefficients are used as an index of the non-error variance as a result of content sampling. Both split-half and coefficient alpha reliability techniques examine the consistency of responses using a single administration of a test. The former produces an internal-consistency measure between two comparable, predetermined halves of the test, while the latter is based on all possible combinations of items. Split-half reliability is often measured by the Spearman-Brown correlation coefficients, while alpha reliability is measured by the Cronbach alpha. The Cronbach alpha is established by the Kuder-Richardson coefficient reliability KR-20 or KR-21 for unweighted items and by numerous other statistics and techniques for weighted items.

A researcher would only want to investigate internal consistency if the test being used includes items that have something in common. This means that the test must have *additive properties* in order to produce meaningful coefficients of consistency. Additive properties imply that items can be summed, with the total resulting in an interpretable value. For example, if a test was designed to ask patients waiting for doctors' appointments about (a) the reason for presentation, (b) previous history, (c) quality of waiting room reception and atmosphere, and (d) transportation used most frequently to attend a physician appointment, it would be pointless to examine internal consistency. Furthermore, internal-consistency tests are meaningful only if it is possible for respondents to complete the entire test. Tests that are time limited, such as speed tests, are designed to limit the number of full completions and therefore cannot make assumptions as to how individuals would have scored if all the items had been answered. Therefore, tests for internal consistency cannot be used here because items appearing later in the test have a higher likelihood of being incomplete than those appearing earlier.

If internal-consistency reliability coefficients are low, this indicates that random or chance errors are large. It may be because the test has too few items or has items included that have little in common. A low reliability coefficient, however, can also indicate a measurement problem. Experts can usually ascertain the reasons for lower than expected coefficients by visually inspecting the test.

## COEFFICIENTS OF STABILITY: TEST-RETEST AND ALTERNATE FORMS RELIABILITY

The test-retest reliability coefficient estimates how much confidence one can have that a test is generalizable over different occasions, by providing an index of the non-error variance in changes in performance between two testing occasions, using the same test each time. It should not be used if the construct under investigation is expected to fluctuate over time: For example, if the test is measuring a disease state that usually resolves spontaneously (e.g., cystitis), test-retest reliability would provide worthless information. It should also not be used if test results improve on a second administration as a result of practice effects. This is particularly a problem in skill acquisition tests and some tests in which rote learning is possible, since an individual may improve as a result of having been previously tested.

To establish test-retest reliability, the targeted test is administered to the same set of individuals twice at a predetermined interval and under the same conditions. It is important that administrations not be in immediate succession, because the resulting reliability coefficient will not provide an adequate index of non-error variance; that is, random fluctuations in performance across occasions will not be measured. Usually the length of time between administrations is 2 weeks; however, if long-range stability is being examined, periods of months or years can be used. The interval selected is dependent on characteristics of the sample and the use of the test. For example, researchers studying children as a target population usually leave a small interval of time between administrations because of the confounding effects of maturation or history. If a test will be used for long-term prediction and the construct is not expected to fluctuate, longer intervals are warranted. For example, a researcher studying personality traits may want to establish long-range test stability. It should be noted that coefficients of stability derived from long-term data are expected to be lower than those derived from the standard short-term data; thus their interpretation is different.

It is because of the potential contamination described above that the alternative-forms reliability coefficient is sometimes used instead. This measure provides an index of the error variance as a result of changes in performance between two testing occasions, using different equivalent tests administered in immediate succession. That is, it measures the temporal stability and consistency of responses to different equivalent items. A word of caution: It is often very difficult to obtain a true equivalent form. Moreover, when researchers develop tests that examine a new construct or measure an established construct in a different way, the identification of a truly parallel form is very difficult. In these cases, the use of alternate-form reliability over test-retest reliability is debatable. Establishing the appropriateness of the parallel form can be accomplished by validation studies on the two forms to ensure that the tests are measuring the same phenomenon. Moreover, the raw scores from the two forms must be able to be converted to the same derived-score scale. When using alternative forms, a low reliability coefficient can be the result of either the use of a nonparallel form, the characteristics of the construct, or a true indication of the nonstability of the construct or instrument.

## INTERRATER RELIABILITY AND EXAMINER RELIABILITY

Interrater reliability and examiner reliability provide indices of error variance that are attributable to scorers and to test administrators, respectively. The former involves having two trained individuals independently score the same test. The degree of this reliability is particularly essential when tests are subject to scorer judgment: for example, assessments evaluating residents' performance. Examiner reliability is estimated by having the same individual complete a test twice, with the instrument being administered by a different individual each time. Particularly, when a study protocol involves interviews, verbal instructions, or the presence of an examiner, researchers are strongly encouraged to consider this form of reliability because if characteristics of the administrator contribute to different results, the repeatability of the measure becomes questionable. Note that since this form of reliability measurement requires two administrations, the limitations of test-retest apply here.

## Validity

Confidence that a test measures what it is intended to measure with the smallest margin of error is only attained by the careful interpretation of its validity. Validity estimates are derived from objective sources of information and by empirical investigations that have been designed to establish what a test measures and how well it measures it. Unfortunately some naive researchers use information from test titles, authors' descriptions, and test prominence to judge the validity of a test, and often incongruence is seen between details derived from these sources and what is being measured.

Critiques may be available on tests under consideration, which will make it easier to judge their validity. Some sources of critiques include Buros (1983, 1985), Grotevant and Carlson (1989), McDowell and Newell (1987), the Test Corporation of America (1986a, 1986b), and Chapter 15 in this book. The researcher may also need to consider newer less prominent tests, however, and these are often not critiqued. In this case a critical appraisal of the published and unpublished data on the test is necessary.

Showing that a test is valid (i.e., truthful) is sometimes straightforward. For example, the mercury manometer reading of blood pressure can be validated through the reading of the arterial blood pressure by an arterial line. Frequently, however, things are more complicated. Consider trying to measure social support, anxiety, or a construct such the "white coat syndrome." Complications arise because of the number of variables that can impinge on accurate measurements, and difficulty in verifying the measurement with some external criterion. It is because of these complications that validity testing is so important.

Validation of a test is an ongoing process. A test is never proven valid once and for all. Each study using the test provides new data to evaluate its validity. For example, newer research may suggest that the test is more useful for some subgroups of patients than others and therefore calls into question the meaningful interpretation of the original estimates as an index of validity.

In addition to being ongoing, validation must be anchored to a specific purpose. A test that has validity for one purpose may not have it for another. Although some popular and well-known tests claim to measure various constructs and traits, none are appropriate for all purposes. Therefore researchers must select a test that is appropriate for their specific situation and that measures what it is they wish to measure with the smallest margin of error. For example, if a researcher examined social support and its effects on the health status of the elderly, using a social support measure that had been validated with single mothers, serious concerns would arise about the validity of the measurement. Not only can the researcher not claim the same psychometric properties, but the validity of the measure may have to be redetermined on a sample that better represents the target population. Another example common in primary care is to use a test designed for screening, such as the Family APGAR (Smilkstein, 1978), as an outcome measure in a study evaluating therapy. No test can be categorized as having any degree of validity without reference to the particular use for which it is being considered, and a test with multiple purposes must have evidence to support each of the claims. When we discuss validity, we are not referring to the measurements but to the use to which the instrument is applied.

The kind of empirical evidence required to make conclusions about each test purpose is contingent on the type of validity being addressed. Validity estimates, however, cannot be based only on an authority's opinion, theory, or mathematical proof; empirical investigations must include evidence from the real world. This is one of the essential concepts of validity.

*Content validity* refers to the sampling adequacy of items in an instrument. *Face validity* examines whether the target population thinks that the instrument measures what it is supposed to measure. *Criterion-related validity* (predictive or concurrent) refers to the degree to which scores on the test are correlated with some external criterion. In predictive criterion-related validity, a future criterion is used, while in concurrent criterion-related validity an existing criterion is used. Finally, construct validity examines the degree to which the items in the test measure the construct under investigation.

## CONTENT AND FACE VALIDITY

Content validation requires the systematic investigation of a test to determine whether its items adequately sample the domain being tested and whether they are constructed in the most appropriate form. Such a procedure is considered part of the plan and construction of a test and therefore is executed before the test is used empirically. It helps address whether scientific generalizations can be made about a specific domain from the items in a test. Content validity should always be examined in the development of any new test, since it allows the researcher to be confident that the test, prior to piloting, is viewed by experts as an adequate measure of what it is supposed to measure.

Face validity refers to what a test superficially measures, not to what it actually measures. It is usually established by asking representatives of the target population whether the proposed instrument *looks* as if it will measure what they understand the construct to be. Face validation is often forgotten and is not a replacement for content validation, but it is an important concept because if the population who will be completing the measure doubt its relevance, the researcher can expect poor response rates and possibly response biases.

Tudiver and Ferris (Chapter 8) discuss some of the more common procedures for establishing both face validity and content validity.

## CRITERION-RELATED VALIDATION

Criterion-related validation requires the empirical investigation of the predictive performance of a test with a predetermined direct and independent outcome. This outcome is measured by a criterion. It is essential that the criterion being used is appropriate and can be measured with the least amount of error. If a test measures what it says it will measure, then it should be highly predictive of the selected criterion. For example, a test that measures medical competence could be validated against an independent measure of performance in clinical practice, to attain an index of how predictive it is of performance. The validation procedure would demonstrate how much one can generalize from the test to the criterion and would provide evidence for the amount of validity in statements of generalizability.

Criterion are of two types: concurrent and predictive. *Concurrent criteria* are outcomes that can be viewed as an immediate substitution of the phenomenon under investigation; *predictive criteria* are outcomes that are available for investigation after a stated period of time. For example, if performance in clinical practice were to be measured immediately after the administering of the test in question, then the criterion would be concurrent; if it were measured 4 years later, the criterion would be predictive. Simultaneous determinations of blood pressure by a mercury manometer and by direct reading through an arterial line is another example of concurrent validity; confirmation of a disease at autopsy is an example of predictive validity.

## CONSTRUCT VALIDATION

Construct validation requires an examination of how well a test measures a theoretical construct. It is frequently quoted but tends to be poorly understood. The problem is that theoretical constructs do not exist as an isolated, observable dimension of behavior (Nunnally, 1978). A construct is something that scientists develop in their own minds to explain and organize observed behavior. For example, the "white coat syndrome," quality of life, intelligence, anxiety, and locus of control are all constructs. The nature of constructs is that they are enduring and abstract. Construct validation involves the use of multiple data sources and multiple investigations, with more evidence for the validity of a construct being offered each time.

Two of the most common ways to investigate construct validity are the factorial approach and the multitrait multimethod approach. In the former, researchers are interested in empirically demonstrating through factor analysis whether discernible underlying theoretical constructs exist. These constructs are established a priori. Items subjected to a factor analysis that measures the same underlying construct should load heavily on the same factor and not load to any great extent on other factors. For example, in a test designed to measure premenstrual syndrome, one would want items asking about symptomology to load on the same factor and not load to any great magnitude with other items on the test that relate to health history, demographics, or self-care practices. Obviously all these areas are important, but items pertaining to each of them should have differential loading.

The multitrait-multimethod approach uses convergent and discriminant evaluations to establish construct validity. *Convergent validation* confirms whether a test correlates with other variables that theoretically measure the same phenomenon; *discriminant validation* confirms that it does not correlate with variables that are *not* considered measurements of the same construct. Construct validation usually involves consideration of both types of data. For example, a test that is said to measure pain perception resulting from an illness should show a high correlation with measures of pain thresholds, but not with common psychiatric syndromes such as hypochondriasis, neurasthenia, and conversion reaction. These validation studies result in the construction of a multitrait-multimethod grid, which is examined for zero-order positive and negative correlations with varying levels of magnitude to establish whether the construct is clearly discernible. Many readers will find it difficult to distinguish between this approach and criterion-related validation. In fact, a great deal of confusion appears in the literature concerning these two methods. Basically, if one chooses to use the multitrait-multimethod approach, some of the results are appropriate to use for both construct and criterion-related validation.

## Reliability, Validity, and Norms

Reliability and validity are not totally independent. While a test may be reliable but not valid, a valid test must have a degree of reliability. Said another way, a test may, on repeated trials, produce the same result but the result may have no validity (truth). For example, a thermometer may consistently show the same reading on repeated trials but be inaccurate; however, a thermometer that closely approximates the correct temperature (i.e., is valid) will always be somewhat reliable. A margin of error can be estimated and is said to be set by the upper and lower boundaries of the confidence interval.

The statistical estimates of reliability and validity are thus related and reflect how reliability limits validity. Technically a validity coefficient (the measure of the validity) cannot exceed the square root of the reliability coefficient (the measure of the reliability). (For example, if the reliability of a test is .80, the test validity cannot exceed .89.) If it does, a sampling error may have occurred and the validity estimate should not be used.

Many tests used in primary care research have established *norms.* Essentially, norms are empirically established frames of reference that represent the average scores of a standardized sample. Test norms are not interpreted as gold standards but rather are translated into the typical or average expected score of individuals similar to those in the representative sample from which the norms were derived. Norms are usually reported in the form of transformed standard scores (linear or normalized) or as percentiles. They may be reported for the full representative sample or for recognizable subgroups. If specific subgroups yield statistically different scores from those in the broadly defined sample, the reporting of norms by subgroups is appropriate. For example, infant and preschool tests often provide norms for each month of age up to the age of 5 or 6.

All norms are restricted to the particular population on which the average scores were derived. Just as validation must be anchored to a specific purpose, the interpretation of normed data must be considered in light of the way the data were obtained and the description of the normative sample. Norms can be derived by a sample that was restricted by age, sex, ethnoracial grouping, education, setting, and so on. The characteristics of the normative sample should be known before scores are compared to these frames of reference. Often primary care researchers are interested in a particular subgroup for which no separately reported norms exist, or they are targeting a population that was never included in the normative sample. In these cases the applicability of the norms to the population being researched must be considered carefully.

Any investigations that aim to establish reliability and validity estimates or norms are subject to the same stringent criteria as those of any other study. That is, attention must be paid to the sampling frame, size of sample, standardized procedures, and statistical analysis. The quality of the research to establish the psychometric properties must be critiqued before confidence can be placed in the results of the studies.

# Magnitude of Reliability and Validity Coefficients

Even in optimal conditions no test is perfectly reliable and valid. Psychometrics provides an indication of the *degree* of these dimensions in an effort to help test users select the most appropriate instrument for their purposes. While one researcher may be satisfied with a particular test's psychometric properties, another may be unwilling to accept them. The decision is often based on the number and kind of conclusions that will be made. For example, if the results of a study will be used to change clinical practice or to establish safe inclusion criteria for enrolling patients in clinical trials, the degree of reliability and validity of the measure will need to be very high. In these instances, consultation with an expert in psychometrics is essential for responsible practice. If, however, a test is simply being used to evaluate satisfaction with services received, the estimates associated with an acceptable test may not need to be more than moderate. Or, if the test is just one of many, the psychometric estimates may not need to be as high as if it were the only measure.

For most research in behavioral medicine, a reliability of at least .80 and a validity of at least .70 seem to represent the basic acceptable estimates. It should be stressed, however, that these values may need to be higher, depending on the types of decisions made and the conclusions derived from a study.

## Conclusion

Any time a test is changed, new reliability and validity estimates need to be established (for more information, see Chapter 9). For example, if a researcher changes a test's face, form, content, presentation of items, scoring, or procedural practices, the original psychometric properties may no longer hold. This possibility poses a major problem to carrying out research and to interpreting research findings. Fully reestablishing the psychometric properties of modified tests is costly and time-consuming, and many researchers do not and, in fact, cannot do so. The issue is further complicated by the fact that even when established tests are used in their original format, they often are applied to populations that differ in many respects from the one that was used originally to establish reliability and validity.

To minimize the errors generated by test modification, population variation, and the like, primary care researchers should seek the advice of an expert in this field during the planning and execution phases of the inquiry. Almost always, compromises may have to be made, and the choice of how to balance between these concessions will affect both the strength and generalizability of the eventual results of the study.

## References

Buros, O. K. (Ed.). (1983). *Tests in print, 111.* Lincoln: University of Nebraska, Buros Institute of Mental Measurements.

Buros, O. K. (Ed.). (1985). *The ninth mental measurements yearbook.* Lincoln: University of Nebraska, Buros Institute of Mental Measurements.

Grotevant, H. D., & Carlson, C. I. (1989). *Family assessments: A guide to methods and measures.* New York: Guilford.

McDowell, I., & Newell, C. (1987). *Measuring health: A guide to rating scales and question- naires.* New York: Oxford University Press.

Nunnally, J. (1978). *Psychometric theory* (2nd ed). New York: McGraw-Hill.

Smilkstein, G. (1978). The family APGAR: A proposal for a family function test and its uses by physicians. *Journal of Family Practice, 6,* 1231-1239.

Test Corporation of America. (1986a). *Test critiques.* Kansas City, MO: Westport.

Test Corporation of America. (1986b). *Tests.* Kansas City, MO: Westport.

# PART TWO

# BASIC TECHNIQUES

## 7 How to Select a Sample in Primary Care Research

TRULS ØSTBYE

In survey research one is often interested in describing the characteristics of a population, usually a large group of people in a defined setting such as a community. For practical reasons, however, one must select a subset of this population—a sample. This chapter addresses the fundamental question: How does one go about selecting a sample that fairly represents the population of interest?

To illustrate the issues explored here, I will present a hypothetical case of a community doctor who wants to carry out a study of obesity in her practice area. Dr. Sheena McKenzie is a physician in Moose Landing, a rural county in Northern Ontario. She has lately observed quite a number of very obese patients in her office. Being interested in nutrition, she wants to confirm whether obesity is a more common problem in Moose Landing than in the rest of Canada and, if so, what are the reasons behind this.

The best study method would be to travel from house to house in Moose Landing and ask everybody to be weighed and measured. To visit everybody would be a truly daunting task, however, so a subset of the population is needed.

## Specifying the Research Question

Dr. McKenzie begins her study by carrying out a literature review and also consulting with colleagues experienced in research. These steps are necessary to assist in formulating a clear research question and developing a study design. Her stated goal is to determine the prevalence of overweight and obese residents in Moose Landing; and secondarily, to explore various factors that may be associated with these problems.

From her literature review, Dr. McKenzie realizes that self-reported information on weight is fraught with problems. Accordingly, she decides that she and a public health nurse will measure the subjects themselves. She also decides to ask her subjects to complete a questionnaire with information relating to food intake, work, physical exercise, and other related issues.

## Determining What to Measure

It is always important to choose a measurement that is valid (does it reflect what the researcher wants to measure?). As a measurement for obesity, one cannot choose weight in itself: A tall man weighing 150 pounds is not obese, but a short woman of the same weight would be. Dr. McKenzie therefore settles on Body Mass Index (BMI): weight in kilograms divided by height in meters squared. This measurement corrects weight for height, is simple to obtain, and has been validated extensively in other studies. It also has been reported in a number of earlier surveys of the whole Canadian population, which gives Dr. McKenzie an opportunity to compare the situation in Moose Landing with that in the rest of the country (bearing in mind that the national norms are not necessarily "normal" in the sense of being optimal from a health point of view). Being overweight is defined as having a BMI of above 25 kilograms per square meter, obesity as a BMI above 30, and morbid obesity as a BMI above 40.

## Population and Sample

A population is the whole collection of units from which a sample may be drawn. In the example, this is all people residing in the county of Moose Landing, covering an area of over 10,000 square kilometers. At the last census (in 1986) the population was determined to be 35,356. Dr. McKenzie realizes that it would be very expensive and time-consuming to survey the entire population, so she determines to select a smaller, representative group of individuals from it—a sample—and use the data derived from this group to make generalizations about the whole. The main criterion when choosing a sample is to ensure that it provides a faithful representation of the totality from which it is selected.

To arrive at such a sample, one must first clearly define the population in terms of three factors: content, extent, and time. An example here could be (a) all individuals (alternatively: all individuals age 15 or over; all Native Canadians), (b) living anywhere in the county of Moose Landing (alternatively: living only in agricultural areas), (c) on May 28, 1991 (alternatively: some other date). These factors are analogous to the conventional terms used to define a population in epidemiological research: person, place, and time.

The population (and sample) is usually, but not necessarily, a defined number of persons (patients, citizens, physicians). The units that make up the population may be institutions (e.g., health centers), families, medical records, biological samples (e.g., urine samples, biopsy material), or events (e.g., office visits or occurrences of coryza, in which cases one individual may contribute one or many events). The unit of interest in the population and the sample is referred to as a *sampling unit*.

An all-too-common source of error is to confuse different sampling units within the same study: for example, to consider encounters rather than individual patients as the sampling unit. In certain studies (e.g., billing studies) the encounter may well be the unit of interest. Here, however, if Dr. McKenzie records that in the past year, 2,000 of her 6,000 visits were by obese patients (thereby implying that one third of residents in Moose Landing are obese), this would be misleading; it is very important to differentiate between 2,000 visits by different patients, and 2,000 visits consisting of 200 patients with an average of 10 visits each.

A particular aspect of the population (for example, the average BMI for men over 30 years of age, or the percentage of women with a BMI over 25) is called a *parameter*; its counterpart in the selected sample is called a *statistic*. The primary objective of sampling theory is to provide accurate estimates of unknown parameters from sample statistics, since these are more easily calculated.

## AN OFFICE-BASED SAMPLE?

It would be simplest for Dr. McKenzie to just work in her office as usual; during each regular clinical encounter, measure the patient's height and weight in a standardized fashion; and then summarize the data she had collected after a certain period of time, say 1 month.

The fundamental problem with this approach (an example of what is called *sequential sampling*) is that the individuals who present in her practice are very likely somehow different from those who do not and thus are likely to be different from the total population of Moose Landing to which she wants to generalize. It is well known that obesity, in its extreme form a disease itself, is also a risk factor for a whole series of other disorders. It is therefore likely that patients tend to be heavier than the general population and thus would not constitute a particularly representative sample.

To further complicate matters, quite a few of her patients come from the neighboring county and thus fall outside her defined population of interest. She is well known for her interest in obesity, and if a physician has a particular training or experience with a particular disease, it is likely that he or she will diagnose that disease more often. This scenario occurs partly because patients with the disease will go out of their way to see someone known to be familiar with it, and partly because such a physician will be particularly observant for symptoms of that disease and may even tend to overdiagnose.

Finally, to add yet another bias—this time in the opposite direction—health problems are not all necessarily *more* common in the office than in the community. Individuals with certain disorders with stigma attached—such as obesity—may tend to avoid professionals whom they rightly or wrongly perceive as unnecessarily judgmental.

In conclusion, for a number of reasons, office-based samples from a general practice are not necessarily representative of the population of interest. They are more likely to be representative if the following criteria are met:

- The practice is alone in a certain district, so that few patients go elsewhere for care.
- The disease is so serious that most individuals would seek help for it.
- The sampling period is long enough (e.g., over 1 year) for most of the population to have been through the physician's office.

## A SAMPLE FROM A WORKPLACE?

Having considered the idea of including only individuals who pass through her own practice, Dr. McKenzie considers the alternative of approaching the Moose Landing Machine Factory to obtain her sample. About 500 people work there, and they come from all over the county. Their ages are quite representative of the community (bearing in mind that children and retired persons would not be included). The factory may well be a good sampling site, a great advantage being that the individuals there will all be in one place. In addition the factory owner is known for his interest in employee health and safety.

Dr. McKenzie again has to consider, however, whether the disorder she is looking at is either more or less common in the factory than in the community at large. Is the particular work that goes on in the factory in any way related to obesity? One might assume overweight to be more of a problem if the factory were producing confectionary or beer, but in this case it is involved in the production of machinery. Another form of bias well known from research in occupational medicine may be more serious: the *healthy worker effect*.

This phenomenon was first observed in early studies of mortality relating to work in certain industries expected to be dangerous to the health of the workers (Wen, Tsai, & Gibson, 1983). Contrary to what was expected, mortality was *lower* in these industries than for the rest of the population. The reason was that in order to be employed in these industries, workers had to be very strong and healthy to begin with. Individuals in poorer health would leave for lighter work or not be hired in the first place.

In the example it could well be that overweight individuals would be less likely to work in the Moose Landing Machine Factory than elsewhere, while the very obese may well be overrepresented among people who do not work at all. Thus, as with her practice population, the staff at the Moose Landing Machine Factory are probably not representative of the overall population.

## A VOLUNTEER SAMPLE?

Next, together with the Victoria Order of Nurses and the Red Cross, Dr. McKenzie plans a Health Fair at the Moose Landing Shopping Mall. She decides that one easy way of selecting a community sample is to set up a Weight and Nutrition Booth and to ask passersby whether they would like to volunteer to get their BMI measured and get some advice on weight and nutrition at the same time.

This is probably not a very good idea. It has been shown in the National Diet-Heart Study (American Heart Association, 1980) that, compared with nonvolunteers, people who volunteer to partake in health studies more frequently

are nonsmokers,
are more concerned about their health,
have a higher level of education,
are employed in professional and skilled jobs,
are Protestant or Jewish,
are living in households with children, and
are active in community affairs.

In the example these factors could be compounded by the fact that the volunteers may be more (or less) likely to have weight problems than those who do not come forward. Both volunteer bias and the healthy worker effect are examples of *selection bias*—error due to systematic differences in characteristics between those who are selected for a study and those who are not. This is a core concept to bear in mind when considering which sample to draw from the population.

## A TRUE COMMUNITY SAMPLE?

The samples discussed above are not very satisfactory, being unrepresentative of the population to various degrees. From a theoretical point of view, what is needed is a truly *random sample*—one that is selected in a way that gives each member of the population an equal chance of being chosen. A random sample has two desirable features: It eliminates bias, and it enables one to determine statistically the reliability of the results.

Random assignment should not be confused with haphazard assignment. Random assignment follows a predetermined plan, which is usually devised with the aid of a table of random numbers. The pattern of assignment may appear haphazard, but this appearance arises from the haphazard nature of random numbers, not from any whim of the investigator in allocating subjects (Last, 1988).

Sampling individuals in a rural community can often be a problem if no complete, up-to-date list of the population is available. (This is less of a problem in Ontario, where such lists are maintained by the provincial health plan.) A complete list of all individuals in the population (the sampling units) is called a *sampling frame.*

Even though the number of individuals selected in a sample would be smaller than the whole population (and thus more feasible for Dr. McKenzie and the public health nurse to visit), they still would be scattered all over the county and necessitate major travel expenses. *Cluster sampling* can overcome these difficulties to some degree. Rather than sampling individuals directly from the total population, one can specify clusters, or grouped units. A cluster might be all persons in a village, city block, or family. In general practice, a cluster may be all patients seen by a specific doctor.

Moose Landing is divided by Statistics Canada into about 40 equally large (in population) enumeration areas, which can be viewed as clusters in the example. Thus the most appropriate strategy for Dr. McKenzie seems to be to select randomly a series of these enumeration areas. Within each cluster she can either include everyone for her study or randomly select a certain number of individuals (*two-stage sampling*).

The cluster sampling method is not always the best: Populations cannot always be divided into natural clusters; and studies using this design are more complex to execute (Cochran, 1977). The point is that none of the different sampling schemes discussed above is inherently superior to the others but depends on the resources available and the exact research question being asked. Simple random sampling, however, is always more efficient for a given total number of subjects than is cluster sampling.

## STRATIFIED SAMPLING

A *stratum* in the research context means a group of study units (in the example, a group of individuals) who are similar or live under similar environmental conditions. The population is divided into groups of study units that are similar. The strata may be very different from each other, but within each stratum the study units are more alike in some respect. After the whole population has been divided into two or more strata, a random selection of study units is taken from each, and the same survey is carried out in all.

The population of Moose Landing can, for example, be divided into five age groups and then a sample drawn from within each stratum. This is particularly relevant if major differences in outcome are expected between the different strata.

## SAMPLE SIZE

Sample size is another important aspect of study design. Dr. McKenzie must consider how large her sample has to be in order to say anything meaningful about the population it is based on. To arrive at an estimate of a satisfactory sample size, she needs to specify

- the expected value of the parameter of interest (e.g., average BMI or percentage with BMI over a certain value)
- the expected variation in this measured trait (the more variation, the larger the sample must be)
- how precise she wants her estimate to be (the more precise, the larger the sample must be)

Sample size calculations are not only necessary for cases in which one wants to make inferences to a population as in the example. They are also commonly performed when comparing two samples for some outcome (e.g., clinical drug trials). The first time a researcher attempts to estimate the necessary sample size for a study, and particularly for complicated designs (e.g., cluster sampling), it is well worth seeking assistance from a more experienced colleague or statistician. (For a good introduction to sample size calculation, see Colton, 1974.)

## QUALITATIVE SAMPLING

This chapter has focused on sampling in *quantitative research*, in which the logic and purpose of quantitative sampling is to select a statistically representative group that permits confident generalization to the larger population.

In the domain of *qualitative research*, the main purpose of sampling is to identify particular information-rich cases and then to study them in great depth. This approach is particularly well suited for exploring research areas in which little is known and the research hypotheses still are quite nonquantitative. A conceptual framework, much less quantifiable parameters, may not yet have been developed.

Qualitative inquiry typically focuses on small samples, selected purposefully. Two examples of purposeful sampling are

- *Extreme case sampling.* These are cases that are extreme in the manifestations of the phenomenon in question. In the example a few extremely obese individuals would be chosen and interviewed in depth, not because they were representative, but because they may illustrate clearly certain issues relating to obesity.
- *Sampling politically important cases.* If it is important to make a study and its results known, one can make a point by including politically important individuals in it. For example, if the mayor of Moose Landing or the editor of the local newspaper is overweight, he or she should be included to give visibility to the study and possibly to make it easier to implement any policy recommendations that may result.

These are just two examples of many qualitative sampling techniques that have been developed. For a discussion of others (homogenous sampling, snowball sampling, typical case sampling, opportunistic sampling, etc.), the reader is referred to Patton (1990).

Qualitative research in general, and qualitative sampling techniques in particular, are not yet commonly used in medical research. If this type of sampling is to be used in a study, it may be prudent to specify explicitly its strengths and limitations when the results are presented.

## Generalizability

When the results of Dr. McKenzie's study are finally available, the question she faces is: To whom can the findings be generalized? The occurrence of obesity is probably quite similar between Moose Landing and other areas in Northern Ontario. The evaluation of *generalizability* (also called *external validity*) goes beyond the data collected in the study and is not just a statistical issue. Judgments about the generalizability of a particular study must involve substantial knowledge of the health problem in question, as well as knowledge of how similar the studied populations is to the one the researcher wants to generalize to.

## Recommendations for Further Reading

Colton (1974) has written a comprehensive introductory biostatistics text, which includes sections on sample size calculation. Leaverton (1986) gives a concise introduction to biostatistics, well suited for self-study. Hulley and Cummings (1988) use clear explanations, tables, and graphics to explain the design of clinical research (little calculus is needed). Norman and Streiner (1986) and Streiner, Norman, and Blum (1989) are in the PDQ (Pretty Darn Quick) series: two slim volumes that give introductions to the fields of biostatistics and epidemiology, respectively. Patton (1990) provides a very readable introduction to qualitative research in general, and qualitative (purposeful) sampling in particular. Many of the definitions of terms used in this chapter are taken from Last (1988).

## References

American Heart Association. (1980). The National Diet-Heart Study: Final report. *American Heart Association Monograph No. 18*. New York: Author.

Cochran, W. G. (1977). *Sampling Techniques*. New York: John Wiley.

Colton, T. (1974). *Statistics in medicine*. Boston: Little, Brown.

Hulley, S. B., & Cummings, S. R. (1988). *Designing clinical research*. Baltimore, MD: Williams and Wilkins.

Last, J. M. (Ed.). (1988). *A dictionary of epidemiology*. New York: Oxford University Press.

Leaverton, P. E. (1986). *A review of biostatistics*. Boston: Little, Brown.

Norman, G. R., & Streiner, D. L. (1986). *PDQ statistics*. Toronto: BC Decker.

Patton, M. Q. (1990). *Qualitative evaluation and research methods* (2nd ed.). Newbury Park, CA: Sage.

Streiner, D. L., Norman, G. R., & Blum, H. M. (1989). *PDQ epidemiology*. Toronto: BC Decker.

Wen, C. P., Tsai, S. P., & Gibson, R. L. (1983). Anatomy of the healthy worker effect: A critical review. *Journal of Occupational Medicine, 25*, 283-289.

# 8 Creating an Original Measure

FRED TUDIVER
LORRAINE E. FERRIS

Chapters 6 and 9 address the importance of using measures that meet the requirements of your specific research purposes and that have known and acceptable reliability and validity properties. When several existing instruments are available, choosing one of these is the initial step. On occasion, however, none will meet your criteria, so you will have to either modify an existing instrument or develop a new one. The first option—making new measures from old—is covered by Zyzanski in Chapter 9. Here we discuss how to develop an original measure: specifically, a self-administered paper-and-pencil questionnaire for use in primary care research.

Developing and validating a new instrument must be conducted in such a way that it will have general appeal to other researchers. Since one of the goals of primary care research is to build a body of knowledge, it is imperative that findings be comparable across studies. This often requires standardized maneuvers, especially in instrumentation. Therefore your instrument will need to be seen as having value for use in other studies. In addition, confidence in the repeatability of your findings is based, at least in part, on the quality of your measure. Therefore the research and clinical communities must regard it as reliable, valid, and functional.

We will restrict the discussion here to the preliminary stages of development of a new measure—the transition from formulating the initial concepts and content to drafting a preliminary form of the instrument. Zyzanski (Chapter 9) and Ferris and Norton (Chapter 6) provide excellent overviews of the later stages of development, including theory and evaluation of psychometric properties.

# Do You Need to Create an Original Measure?

It is in a researcher's best interest to use an existing instrument whenever possible. Creating an original one is expensive and time-consuming—we estimate the average time commitment required for creating, initially testing, and evaluating a 45- to 75-item measure to be at least 1-2 years. Thus, as in modifying an old instrument, the decision to create a new one is not to be taken lightly.

As you progress through the fundamental stages of developing the purpose, conceptual framework, hypotheses or questions, and design of your project, the requirements for the measure will come to be identified, along with the necessary information to evaluate whether any appropriate instruments already exist. Such information includes carefully considering who the target population will be, how and where the measure will be administered, how the data will be analyzed, and what statistical conclusions will be sought based on the analysis. For example, a survey completed postoperatively in a hospital by cardiac surgery patients will necessarily be very different from one mailed to people at high risk for cardiovascular disease; similarly, an instrument whose purpose is to screen potential migraine patients for a clinical trial cannot be used to evaluate the effectiveness of interventions for the same condition.

You may take several steps to safeguard against the unnecessary development of an original measure. First, perform a computerized search of data sources for germane research, and note the measures used. Searching such resources as *Medline, Index Medicus, Psychological Abstracts, Behavioral Medicine Abstracts,* and *Education Abstracts* will result in the identification of relevant research and editorials. Some of these articles will appear in journals known for publishing instrument development papers, including though not limited to *American Journal of Public Health, Journal of Abnormal and Social Psychology, Journal of Applied Behavior Science, Journal of Behavioral Medicine, Journal of Clinical Psychology, Journal of Community Health, Journal of Health and Social Behaviour, Journal of Medical Education, Journal of Personality and Social Psychology, Medical Care, Preventive Medicine, Sociometry,* and *Social Science and Medicine.*

Second, review reference books that specialize in listing and reviewing available measures. This stage serves two purposes: to cross-validate the list of measures you identified through your search of the literature, and to provide critical reviews of those that seem like possibilities. Such books include those published by the Buros Institute of Mental Measurements and the Test Corporation of America. Two popular books that review measures suitable for primary care researchers are those by Grotevant and Carlson (1989) and McDowell and Newell (1987).

## Advantages and Disadvantages of Creating an Original Measure

Creating your own measure, as opposed to using an existing one in either original or modified form, has several advantages. First and foremost, it will emanate from your own particular theory and conceptual framework, not someone else's. Second, it will focus on addressing your research questions and so will not contain extraneous items. This focus will increase its content and face validity and also yield higher construct validity estimates. Third, it will be devised and pretested with your target population, guaranteed to be chosen from patients with diseases or conditions, ethnoracial backgrounds, health history, and other characteristics representative of your target population. Fourth, it will meet your own structure and administration specifications. For example, if you intend to use it as one in a battery of questionnaires to be completed in a busy clinic setting, you do not want to be restricted to following the requirements of an existing measure that may include a long administration.

Disadvantages exist as well, however. First, as mentioned previously, creating an original measure requires much time, energy, and often, money. It may take several years to test on targeted populations and settings and by different teams of researchers, and during this time the study of the research question is at an impasse. For urgent clinical studies this standstill is inappropriate. Second, it requires a degree of expertise that is often beyond the scope of most clinical primary care researchers and usually beyond the reach of available resources.

## Stages in the Creation of an Original Measure

The creation of an original measure has six stages:

1. Identifying and prioritizing content areas
2. Generating items for each content area
3. Quantifying selected items
4. Determining the content and face validity

5. Final review of items
6. Formatting the new measure

These are discussed in turn below.

### 1. *Identifying and prioritizing content areas.*

Conceptual perspectives and theoretical underpinnings will direct the identification of content areas or domains, as well as the relative importance of each. Incorporating one's own opinions is important; however, this should by no means be the only source. A review of other studies usually will assist in these tasks. For example, a review of studies using the health-belief model will demonstrate that it is well defined.

An additional approach is to arrange for a panel of experts in the relevant clinical or research area to help choose and prioritize content areas or domains. Ideally these individuals should also have skills in instrument development.

Choose this panel very carefully. One method is to ask several professionals in the primary care field to independently generate lists of people whom they consider to be experts in the area of study; then approach those whose names appear repeatedly. Another method is to do a citation search of the authors identified in your literature review and to approach those most frequently cited. Unfortunately clinicians may be overlooked in this process because these individuals often do not publish. Useful sources for finding clinician experts are specialized clinics, academic clinical settings, and sites of clinical trials.

It is usually advisable to include also a panel of people who may be representative of the proposed study population in helping to identify content areas. Individuals who participate in the stages of instrument development should not later be included in the study, so if the target population is small, this may not be feasible.

Have the expert panel generate content areas through independent or group work. Sometimes it is best if they execute the task independently and then meet to reach a consensus; sometimes they should work together from the start: The choice is often a pragmatic one, based on time commitment, distances, and the number of people involved. If group work is required at all, use systematic procedures to elicit the information. One such procedure is the nominal group technique (Delbecq, Van de Ven, & Gustafson, 1975), which employs a group process method to elicit first independent and then group opinions on a specific topic. This technique is appealing because it overcomes common problems of group dynamics, especially the monopolization of time by a few members.

Another useful technique is the focus group, discussed in depth in Chapter 15 by David Morgan.

All reports generated from the research study should describe carefully the identification and prioritizing process. Include a full description of the panels, your selection procedures, and the methods employed to produce the information.

## 2. *Generating items for each content area.*

Generate a large pool of items for each content area, enough to sample it adequately. The actual number of items should be determined by the relative importance of the dimension: The minimal number per content area should probably be not less than 10. Subsequent steps will result in the elimination of some items, so it is advisable that you initially include all items, even those that could be outliers.

The process of trying to write specific questions for a content area helps clarify the research purpose and the operational definition of the content area. Ambiguities in the wording of questions or alternative ways of asking them highlight the need to reevaluate how an item relates to other items in the content area and to the overall content domain. For every item generated, the constructor should demonstrate its relationship with other content-similar items and to the overall purpose of the study. Often a constructor will include questions that would be "interesting to know," only to discover that he or she has jeopardized valid results because these items are not directly relevant to the study.

Be mindful of some major issues when writing items, including how to word nonthreatening questions, questions about sensitive topics, and knowledge and attitude questions. Another issue is whether questions should be open- or closed-ended. Open-ended questions do not provide response options: For example, "What is the most upsetting symptom you are experiencing?" or "What do you think is the most serious problem your family has to deal with concerning your illness?" Closed-ended questions require that the respondent select one or more predetermined response options: For example, "Do you take your medication as directed by your physician: yes or no?" "Which of the following people do you routinely see in this clinic: physician, nurse, social worker, psychologist, occupational therapist?" Several books address these and other major issues (see for example, Dillman, 1978; Sudman & Bradburn, 1983), and we strongly recommend that test constructors consult them.

## 3. *Quantifying selected items.*

Special techniques exist for devising the possible answers to closed-ended questions in order to allow you to characterize, categorize, or evaluate individuals or groups with as much discriminating power as necessary. Your choice of possible answers will dictate the level of measurement that your new instrument will achieve: nominal, ordinal, interval, or ratio. David Wilkin (Chapter 5) discusses this issue in more depth. Additional references that should be consulted include books on instrument construction (see for example, Bennett & Ritchie, 1975; Del Greco & Walop, 1987a; Dillman, 1978; Payne, 1951; Woodward & Chambers, 1986) and instrument design (see for example, Del Greco & Walop, 1987b; Del Greco, Walop, & Eastridge, 1987a, 1987b; Dillman, 1978; Oppenheim, 1966; Sudman & Bradburn, 1983).

In general, quantification of an item will be dependent on how amenable it is to certain response options. Closed-ended questions may be best answered by yes-no, multiple choice, or scales. For example, we recommend using yes-no answers to record the symptoms a patient is experiencing. Multiple-choice questions are useful both for measuring knowledge and for other types of questions: For example, "What do you think is the most effective birth control method?" (list methods and respondent selects one) or "While waiting for your appointment, which of the following activities do you engage in?" (list activities and respondent checks all that apply) or "Which of the following statements most reflects how you feel?" (list options and respondents check one or more). Scaled questions are often used to assess attitudes: for example, "A woman should have a breast examination annually" (strongly agree, agree, disagree, strongly disagree). Test constructors need to decide whether to provide such options as don't know, no opinion, undecided, or no answer. The alternative is forced-choice questions, which require respondents to select one alternative that is closest to their answer; provisions for "sitting on the fence" are not available.

### 4. *Determining the content and face validity.*
After quantifying items, the researcher should examine the content and face validity of the research questions to ensure that the planned statistical analysis will produce meaningful results. Unlike other types of validity that examine the properties of a measure after its construction and administration to the target population, these are assessed during the development stage. Content validity requires a systematic examination of whether the test items adequately sample the specific domain and whether they are constructed in the most appropriate form to test the content area. Face validity refers to whether the instrument appears, on the surface, to measure what it purports to, rather than what it actually measures. Face validity is not a replacement for content validity, but it must be established because if it is lacking, you may expect poor response

rates, and possibly, response biases. Ferris and Norton (Chapter 6) provide a detailed description of content and face validity.

Both these types of validation require systematic investigations, with that for content occurring first. Experts in the relevant field should be asked to examine the measure for content validity. *Consensual validation* refers to the process of getting more than one opinion. It is best if these individuals are different from those used to identify and prioritize the content areas (see Step 1 for suggestions on how to recruit and employ experts). Provide them with as much information as they need to evaluate whether the instrument adequately samples the content area. At the very least, this information should include a written description of the research purpose, conceptual framework, research hypotheses or questions, research design, description of target population, and planned statistical analyses. You may increase the response rate if you also inform them of your selection process, why others cannot replace them, and what contribution their participation will make. For the investigation of face validity, it is more important to have several members from the target population examine the measure, although the experts may be asked to do this as well.

The information obtained from this process can be recorded either quantitatively or qualitatively to determine content and face validity. In our experience we have found a combination of these strategies to be most useful.

When relevancy and clarity are asssessed on a 5-point Likert scale, a minimum of 10 experts is required in order for relevancy and clarity scores for an item to be calculated. The variance and means of their responses are used to determine whether these scores are acceptable. Low variance indicates agreement, while the mean shows the direction of that agreement.

Establish cutoff values for acceptability before analyzing the responses. For example, since the maximum score on a 5-point scale is 4 and the minimum zero, an acceptable level could be a variance of .6 or lower. A cutoff value for an acceptable mean on a 5-point scale would be at least a 3 (moderate level). Both of these decisions depend of course on the purpose of your instrument. Eliminate items that fail to reach an acceptable relevancy score; reword those that reach an acceptable relevancy score but do not meet the criteria for clarity; and retain unchanged those that meet both. Finally, if an item has overall relevance but fails to have relevance to the content area, collect responses to open-ended questions and examine these qualitative data to determine whether a more relevant content area exists for it. For example, items originally assigned to a content area that measures proficiency may be more appropriately allocated to one that measures knowledge.

Open-ended questions about length of the questionnaire, balance of questions, and order of subsections reflect face validity. They are essential for the prioritization of the content areas, as well as for the resolution of some other important instrument design concerns. For example, do the experts believe that the titles for content areas should be on the final measure? Should item order be randomized? These questions are more reflective of face validity than content validity.

After deleting or rewording items, carry out a face validation of the measure, using representative members of the target population. Here the question to ask is: "At first glance, do you feel that this instrument measures what it purports to measure: yes or no?"

If changes are made following the content and face validation, the revised instrument must be resubmitted to a new set of experts or representatives of the target population. In these instances, carry out the content and face validation procedures again.

## 5. Final review of the items.

Examine the revised measure for its readability. Computer software packages are available that can quickly determine the "Fog Index" of your questionnaire, an assessment of what level of education respondents would have to have in order to complete it. For most measures, you will find that an equivalence of eighth grade is probably the highest that can be assumed. If the reading level of the instrument is determined to be higher than that expected in your target population, revise the instrument and resubmit it to the content-validation experts again to ensure that it still measures what it purports to measure.

Finally ask five to ten new people from the target population to fill out the questionnaire. (If the study has a repeated measures design, we suggest you administer the measure the same number of times and under the same conditions as specified in the research.) Note whether they complete it, answer the appropriate items, follow directions appropriately, and how long it takes them. Also ask them about the experience of completing the measure. Any concerns raised should be discussed with the panels of validators.

## 6. Formatting the new measure.

It is now time to design the physical format of the instrument. Researchers often (consciously or not) give the highest priority to meeting their data processing needs, but the respondent's needs should come first. Poorly designed formats of self-administered surveys may result in incomplete or missed responses, incorrect or unreliable responses, or reduced compliance, all of which diminish the reliability and validity of the instrument. We recommend two books on formatting surveys: Dillman (1978), and Sudman and Bradburn (1983). Briefly, we have found the most important elements to consider to be (a) the overall appearance, (b) the layout of question items, (c) the size and format of the text, (d) the format of multiple-choice questions and "skip instructions," and (e) the placement of demographic questions. These are discussed in turn below.

## Overall Appearance

Many survey writers overlook the physical appearance of their instrument, focusing most of their time and effort on its content. Research shows, however, that respondents are more likely to complete a self-administered survey if it has a professional look. This look includes the date, title of the study, and name and logo of the sponsoring organization on the cover. In addition, Dillman (1978) recommends using a booklet form and, if appropriate, reducing the size. A booklet form facilitates reading and answering, makes losing pages less likely, and looks more professional. Desktop publishing software now makes the process of creating professional-looking surveys available to most researchers.

## Layout of Question Items

A haphazard arrangement of items may jeopardize an otherwise well-designed survey. Although the individual items may be in the appropriate content section and in the proper sequence, research shows that optimal response reliability requires their arrangement in specific ways. The following are important general rules to follow:

1. Number the items and allow ample space between them.
2. Do not split an item between two pages; this often leads to confusion and incomplete responses.
3. Do not try to cram as many items as possible on a page to save space or to shorten the perceived length of the instrument, as this will often reduce reliability and increase the amount of missing information in your data. You are better off leaving substantial space for open-ended questions.

## Size and Format of the Text

For reasons mentioned above, many survey writers use small font sizes and/or difficult-to-read text. We have found that a minimum font size of 12 characters per inch (cpi) (*after* any photographic reduction) is sufficient for most surveys; if many of your respondents are over 65 years of age, use at least 10 cpi. The quality of the type is also important. The type quality on most dot matrix printers is not acceptable for self- administered surveys. Use a good-quality laser printer or a professional typesetter for crisp, clear text.

### Format of Multiple-Choice Questions and "Skip Instructions"

Multiple-choice formats are often confusing to respondents. To avoid confusion, place the choices vertically rather than horizontally, and use parallel columns with horizontal headings to facilitate the layout of multiple response items and scaled questions.

Skip instructions (e.g., "If YES then go to question 11") should be used carefully. To avoid respondents' missing the directions, place them *after the answer* and not after the question. In addition, skip instructions should be after a yes response, not after a no response: Sudman and Bradburn (1983) suggest that more errors are made to skips triggered by a no response.

### Placement of Demographic Questions

Virtually all surveys used by primary care researchers contain at least some routine demographic items. Tradition has dictated their placement at the start, but Dillman (1978) makes a plea for locating them at the end. His reason is simple: Most respondents find these questions tedious, and so placing them at the end may ensure that your respondents get past the start of the survey and complete it.

## Summary

Creating an original measure is expensive and time-consuming. If no adequate instrument exists, however, researchers may need to embark on the process. It is essential that constructors of new measures carefully follow each of the stages outlined in this chapter and do not attempt to skip or eliminate steps in the interests of saving time or resources. An instrument will be regarded as a valuable measure when documentation exists affirming the use of a linear and quality process in its development.

# References

Bennett, A. C., & Ritchie, K. (1975). *Questionnaires in medicine: A guide to their design and use*. London: Oxford University Press.

Del Greco, L., & Walop, W. (1987a). Questionnaire development: 1. Formulation. *Canadian Medical Association Journal, 136*, 583-585.

Del Greco, L., & Walop, W. (1987b). Questionnaire development: 5. The pretest. *Canadian Medical Association Journal, 136*, 1025-1026.

Del Greco, L., Walop, W., & Eastridge, L. (1987a). Questionnaire development: 3. Translation. *Canadian Medical Association Journal, 136*, 817-818.

Del Greco, L., Walop, W., & Eastridge, L. (1987b). Questionnaire development: 4. Preparation for analysis. *Canadian Medical Association Journal, 136*, 927-928.

Delbecq, A. L., Van de Ven, A. H., & Gustafson, D. H. (1975). *Group techniques for program planning: A guide to nominal group and delphi processes*. Glenview, IL: Scott, Foresman.

Dillman, D. A. (1978). *Mail and telephone surveys: The total design method*. Toronto: John Wiley.

Grotevant, H. D., & Carlson, C. I. (1989). *Family assessment: A guide to methods and measures*. New York: Guilford.

McDowell, I., & Newell, C. (1987). *Measuring health: A guide to rating scales and questionnaires*. New York: Oxford University Press.

Oppenheim, A. N. (1966). *Questionnaire design and attitude measurement*. New York: Basic Books.

Payne, S. L. (1951). *The art of asking questions*. Princeton, NJ: Princeton University Press.

Sudman, S., & Bradburn, N. M. (1983). *Asking questions: A practical guide to questionnaire design*. San Francisco: Jossey-Bass.

Woodward, C. A., & Chambers, L. W. (1986). *Guide to questionnaire construction and question writing*. Ottawa: Canadian Public Health Association.

# 9 Cutting and Pasting
New Measures From Old

STEPHEN J. ZYZANSKI

In general, cutting and pasting a new measure from an old one is not a strategy to be taken lightly. This is especially true if the planned modifications significantly alter the psychometric properties of the original measures. Once major changes have been made, one can no longer assume that the modified measure is reliable and valid just because the original was shown to have these properties. Thus it is incumbent on the investigator to document the psychometric properties of the modified measure. The success of most studies is dependent on the quality of the data gathered by its measures: A poorly designed or evaluated measure can easily invalidate a study's findings. Reestablishing the psychometric properties of a modified measure will increase confidence in results relating to this measure.

Measures may be modified in a variety of ways. The following four ways are among the most common. First, items from an existing measure are often deleted, either because they are inappropriate for the study population or because the original measure is too long relative to the space limitations of the study. Second, inappropriate items are deleted and newly written ones are added in order to enhance a measure's relevance for a specific study population. Third, aspects of two or more measures are combined to form a composite measure. The separate measures may be used in their entirety or only in part. Fourth, the use of measures that have been developed on one type of population but administed to an entirely new one. An example would be measures developed and standardized on college students but now applied to a geriatric population. In all four of these situations the resulting measure's psychometric properties are unknown. Thus one needs to proceed in a similar fashion to that employed for new instruments; that is, establish the psychometric properties of the reconstituted measure.

The basic building blocks of any measure or scale are the individual items in its makeup. Therefore a measure's success is greatly dependent on the quality of its items. A measure may be accurately described as a "good" measure if it is reliable, valid, and discriminating. In addition it should have good norms and be well tailored to its subjects. These characteristics can be built into measures by sound scale construction.

In creating new measures from old, adhering to these principles will improve the precision and accuracy of measurement. In the following sections the procedures used to get information about scale items are described, along with the procedures used to select items so as to compose the most suitable measure for a given purpose. The relationship of item characteristics to the resulting scale characteristics will also be discussed in regard to the aim of developing a reliable, valid, and discriminating measure.

## Properties of Measures

The characteristics of measures covered in this chapter are dimensionality (factor analysis), item analysis (item-total correlation), reliability (internal consistency and stability over time), validity (concurrent, predictive, and construct), norms, and replication. These characteristics tell how a measure was developed and how well it performs in specific contexts. A well-documented measure will have empirical evidence for each of these characteristics.

Thus one needs first to establish whether the items measure one or multiple dimensions. Once this is established, an item analysis can be conducted separately for each dimension.

After the items are selected, the measure's internal-consistency reliability is calculated. If the measure is designed to assess a stable, traitlike attribute, its stability over time should be examined. It is essential to establish a unidimensional measure's internal-consistency reliability prior to proceeding with validity testing: If it has inadequate reliability, mathematically it can be shown that it cannot exhibit a high correlation with an outcome measure (Guilford, 1954). If it is reliable, however, the process of establishing its validity follows.

Measures are not valid in the abstract but only valid for a specific purpose. Thus, depending on the outcome criterion and the type of study design, evidence of the measure's concurrent or predictive validity is evaluated next. Based on theory and evidence from a variety of sources, a case is built for construct validity; that is, a network of associations that support the contention that the measure actually measures the attribute or dimension in question.

Once some evidence of validity is available, one can begin the process of developing norms for the measure. Norms are based on the mean and standard deviation of the scores in the standardizing population. The larger and more heterogeneous this population, the more likely that the norms will generalize to other, similar study populations. The norms include how the measure is scored, what constitutes a large or small value, and what cutting score best optimizes the discrimination of criterion groups.

The final step in the process involves replicating the item analysis, reliability assessment, and validity determination on an independent sample of subjects. Often study samples are split into two halves and the second half is used to cross-validate the findings from the first. Since the statistical procedures used in scale construction capitalize on chance variation at several steps in the process, it is expected that some shrinkage in reliability and validity will occur. The estimates derived from the new, independent sample are the ones most likely to represent the measure's performance in other studies, not the inflated ones derived from the initial sample. (For more on scaling, see Chapter 5. For more detail on psychometric properties, see Chapter 6.)

## Methods of Item Analysis

The core of any scale construction is the item analysis procedure, which guides in selecting the best items for a scale. Through item analysis all possible items are subjected to a stringent series of evaluation procedures, both individually and within the context of the whole measure. Once these are completed, a great deal is known about the items, including those that do not contribute. Based on the purpose of the scale, items are selected that will maximize the measure's ability to discriminate subjects across the full range of the attribute being measured. Three of the most common methods of scale construction are based on item analyses that are either designed to maximize a scale's internal-consistency reliability, designed to maximize its criterion-related validity, or are derived from factor analysis (Allen & Yen, 1979). For unidimensional scales, the most common method is that designed to maximize reliability. This is probably the single best method to learn, and it applies equally well in the case of scales derived from factor analysis. In this chapter the greatest emphasis will be given to this approach.

One starts this approach by considering four basic criteria for item selection: scale length, scale content, item-total correlation, and discrimination level (Kline, 1986). For length, good reliability is usually achieved with about 20 to 30 items. In terms of content, it is desirable to have as wide a range and variety of items as possible. The higher the item-total correlation, the better the item. Finally the discrimination level is satisfactory if the dichotomized item displays skewness between 20% and 80%.

Several indices may be used for calculating the item-total correlations: point-biserial correlation, phi coefficient, and the Pearson product-moment correlation. For dichotomous items the point biserial is best if the total score is continuous, while the phi coefficient is best if the total score is dichotomized, for example, above or below the mean. If the items are multipoint items and the total score continuous, the Pearson correlation is likely to be best.

A program in the Statistical Package for the Social Sciences (SPSS) is called RELIABILITY and has all of the information necessary for a complete item analysis. Table 9.1 illustrates the nature of the output that this program provides (Nie, Hull, Jenkins, Steinbrenner, & Bent, 1975). The data displayed here are 16 of the 25 items from Hudson's Index of Family Relations administered to 140 pregnant women in a family practice center. The critical information is contained in the last three columns. The corrected item-total correlations tell how each item correlates with a sum composed of the remaining (n-l) items. This is the single most useful statistic in the table; from this column, items for the final scale will be selected. Note in this example that all of the items show a corrected correlation with the total score of at least 0.60, indicating that no poor items are in the pool. The next column displays the squared multiple correlation of each item with the rest of the items. This is a measure of an item's *multicollinearity*, or redundancy. The lower the correlation, the less that item has in common with the others. Items with low correlations would also be candidates to be dropped. The final column represents the internal-consistency reliability coefficient (specifically, Cronbach's alpha statistic) for the remainder of the scale when the item of interest is deleted (Bohrnstedt, 1969). This is yet another marker to use in selecting items. If the scale's reliability is higher without a particular item than with it, that item should be deleted. In this instance the scale's reliability remains high throughout; thus one could probably drop some items and still retain a high level of reliability (over 0.80). This is an important consideration for study protocols that are already too long. Finally, Table 9.1 displays the scale's overall reliability at the bottom, and the relevant scale statistics of mean, range, and variance at the top. The standardized item alpha would be used if the items in the scale were a mixture of response formats. In this case all items were administered in a 5-point response format.

## Item Selection to Maximize a Measure's Reliability

The actual step-by-step procedure for selecting items to maximize a scale's overall reliability is well described in the literature, for example, in the texts by Nunnally (1978) or Kline (1986). The basic steps based on Kline are as follows: In *Step 1* the researcher selects items that meet the two statistical criteria of item-total correlation and item discrimination (the percentage of subjects selecting one response choice). Items near 0% or 100% add little to the total score. Since one purpose of a measure is to spread out individuals along a continuum, the greater the spread achieved, the greater the scale's total variance. Items with large correlations with other items and having large variances themselves will make the greatest contribution to the total scale variance (Rust & Golombok, 1982). Thus the aim is to select only those items that make a large contribution to the total score (item-total correlation) and also display item discrimination levels generally in the range 20% to 80%.

In *Step 2* items that fail one of the two item characteristics criteria are reviewed to see whether any particular characteristics of the sample (e.g., gender, age) could account for this failing. These items will be needed should the scale fall short of its desired reliability level.

In *Step 3* the content of the items selected to this point is inspected. If the range of desired behaviors has not been covered, the unselected items are reviewed for any that may have borderline item characteristics but address the needed content; these can be added to the scale.

In *Step 4* the scale's Cronbach reliability is computed for the items selected. If the reliability is at least 0.7 or at the desired level, the item analysis can be stopped. If the desired reliability has not been achieved, the process is continued by adding new items, and the reliability is reevaluated until the appropriate level has been achieved or the item pool exhausted.

In *Step 5* the distribution of the scores is examined, assuming the item analysis was successful. If the distribution is greatly skewed, steps can be taken to correct it (new items added or the data transformed). The variance should also be as large as possible, indicating that the scale is discriminating well. Assuming the variance is adequate, Ferguson's delta statistic is often computed next (Ferguson, 1949, 1981). This statistic is a

**Table 9.1** Sample Output from SPSS Reliability Program

| Item Statistics Mean | Minimum | Maximum | Range | Max/Min | Variance |
|---|---|---|---|---|---|
| 4.113 | 3.400 | 4.571 | 1.171 | 1.345 | 0.103 |

| Item-Total Statistics | Scale Mean If Item Deleted | Scale Variance If Item Deleted | Corrected Item-Total Correlation | Squared Multiple Correlation | Alpha If Item Deleted |
|---|---|---|---|---|---|
| Item  1 | 61.421 | 177.584 | 0.750 | 0.708 | 0.941 |
| Item  2 | 61.450 | 177.990 | 0.732 | 0.699 | 0.941 |
| Item  3 | 61.686 | 175.915 | 0.704 | 0.634 | 0.942 |
| Item  4 | 61.428 | 182.160 | 0.598 | 0.524 | 0.944 |
| Item  5 | 61.236 | 182.944 | 0.611 | 0.503 | 0.943 |
| Item  6 | 61.736 | 172.484 | 0.813 | 0.743 | 0.939 |
| Item  7 | 61.721 | 171.066 | 0.800 | 0.813 | 0.939 |
| Item  8 | 62.407 | 171.524 | 0.613 | 0.519 | 0.945 |
| Item  9 | 61.879 | 170.410 | 0.774 | 0.718 | 0.940 |
| Item 10 | 61.450 | 182.192 | 0.637 | 0.492 | 0.943 |
| Item 11 | 61.593 | 175.193 | 0.630 | 0.604 | 0.943 |
| Item 12 | 62.121 | 172.856 | 0.636 | 0.569 | 0.944 |
| Item 13 | 61.521 | 174.755 | 0.804 | 0.720 | 0.940 |
| Item 14 | 61.593 | 172.416 | 0.815 | 0.767 | 0.939 |
| Item 15 | 62.236 | 171.462 | 0.736 | 0.587 | 0.941 |
| Item 16 | 61.629 | 176.408 | 0.671 | 0.591 | 0.942 |

RELIABLITY Cofficients ($N=140$), 16 items

◄Alpha = 0.945                      Standardized Item Alpha = 0.948

measure of the discriminating power of the scale; values beyond 0.9 indicate that it is discriminating well across the continuum.

In *Step 6* the entire item analysis should be cross-validated on a new sample. If some items fail the statistical criteria of item- total correlation and item discrimination, they will have to be rewritten and tested again or dropped if the scale has sufficient items.

## Factors Influencing a Measure's Reliability

Since a heavy emphasis is placed on scale construction that maximizes a measure's internal-consistency reliability, several additional factors need to be considered. The first concerns the size of the observed point-biserial correlation. With continuous total scores, this correlation has a curtailed range and can never go beyond 0.8. As the discrimination of the items becomes less, the range of possible values for the correlation

**Table 9.2** Changes in the Reliability Coefficient as a Function of Increasing the Number of Items in a Scale

| Original reliability | Number of times a scale is increased | | | | | | | | |
|---|---|---|---|---|---|---|---|---|---|
| | 2 | 3 | 4 | 5 | 6 | 7 | 8 | 9 | 10 |
| .10 | .18 | .25 | .31 | .36 | .40 | .44 | .47 | .50 | .53 |
| .30 | .46 | .56 | .63 | .68 | .72 | .75 | .77 | .79 | .81 |
| .50 | .67 | .75. | .80 | .83 | .86 | .88 | .89 | .90 | .91 |
| .70 | .82 | .88 | .90 | .92 | .93 | .94 | .95 | .95 | .96 |
| .90 | .95 | .96 | .97 | .98 | .98 | .98 | .99 | .99 | .99 |

Source: Adapted from Ghiselli and Brown, 1955.

becomes even less (Thorndike, 1982). The discrimination not only affects the maximum possible value but also, proportionately, all values less than the maximum. Thus if the correlation in the underlying population is really 0.5 but the responses for a dichotomized item are 25% and 75%, the maximum correlation possible is only 0.36. This truncated range for the point biserial means that one should not be discouraged with lower correlations; they are to be expected. Nunnally (1978), for example, recommends that all items with a corrected item-total correlation of 0.2 be eligible for inclusion in the final scale.

A second issue involving reliability concerns the number of items in a scale. The magnitude of Cronbach's alpha varies as a function of the number of items and the average inter-item correlation. A higher reliability can be achieved by increasing the number of items when inter-item correlations are low. In fact, formulas exist that enable one to calculate how many items would need to be added to a scale to increase the reliability to a desired level (Edwards, 1970). Using the general Spearman-Brown formula

$$R_{kk} = \frac{k\, R_{xx}}{1 + (k-1)\, R_{xx}}$$

where $k$ is the number of items in the lengthened scale divided by the number of items in the base scale, $R_{xx}$ is the reliability of the base test, and $R_{kk}$ is the reliability of the lengthened scale, the values in Table 9.2 illustrate the effect of increasing the number of items on a scale's reliability. For example, if a scale of any length had a reliability of 0.50, then to achieve a reliability of 0.80 one would have to increase its items fourfold. Specifically, if a 10-item scale had a reliability of 0.50, it would require 40 items to increase this reliability to 0.80. Table 9.2 is useful because it shows that if a measure has a low initial reliability, the number of additional items needed to increase its reliability to an adequate level may be too large to be practical.

**Table 9.3** Reduction in the Range of Scores upon the Reliability Coefficient

Decreased range as a % of the total range

| Reliability of the total range | 90% | 80% | 70% | 60% | 50% |
|---|---|---|---|---|---|
| .90 | .88 | .84 | .80 | .72 | .60 |
| .70 | .63 | .53 | .39 | .19 | .00 |
| .50 | .38 | .22 | .00 | .00 | .00 |
| .30 | .14 | .00 | .00 | .00 | .00 |
| .10 | .00 | .00 | .00 | .00 | .00 |

Source: Adapted from Ghiselli and Brown, 1955.

A third issue influencing reliability is the range of individual differences in the attribute or performance of the study sample. As this range becomes smaller, the reliability coefficient decreases. If the reliability is being determined on a group whose range of the attribute is less than that of the total group on which the measure is to be used, the reliability coefficient will be an underestimate. The lower the reliability, the more it will decrease if computed on a reduced range (Gulliksen, 1950). The values in Table 9.3 illustrate this point and are based on the following dispersion formula:

$$R_{uu} = 1 - \frac{S_k^2 (1 - R_{kk})}{S_u^2}$$

where $R_{uu}$ is the unknown population reliability, $S_k^2$ is the variance in the total population or for which the reliability is known, $R_k$ is the known reliability, and $S_u^2$ is the variance of the reduced range for which the reliability is unknown. For example, if the upper 10% and the lower 10% of a population distribution were not included in the analysis of reliability, then the range would be 20% less than that of the total range. If the reliability coefficient of this reduced group was 0.53, then the reliability for the total group would most likely be 0.70.

The final issue regarding reliability concerns its relationship with validity. The extent to which a particular independent measure can correlate with an outcome measure is limited by its own reliability and by that of the outcome to be predicted (Carmines & Zeller, 1979). The values shown in Table 9.4 are based on the following correction for attention formula:

$$R_{xy}^* = \frac{R_{xy}}{\sqrt{R_{xx} \, R_{yy}}}$$

where $R_{xy}^*$ is the expected correlation when both variables are perfectly correlated, $R_{xy}$ is the observed correlation between variables $x$ and $y$, and $R_{xx}$ and $R_{yy}$ are the reliabilities of variables $x$ and $y$. Thus if the reliability

**Table 9.4** Maximum Possible Validity Coeffecient for an Independent Variable Given its Reliability and the Reliability of the Dependent Variable

|  | Reliability of dependent variable | | | | | |
|---|---|---|---|---|---|---|
| Reliability of independent variable | .00 | .20 | .40 | .60 | .80 | 1.00 |
| .00 | .00 | .00 | .00 | .00 | .00 | .00 |
| .20 | .00 | .20 | .28 | .35 | .40 | .45 |
| .40 | .00 | .28 | .40 | .49 | .57 | .63 |
| .60 | .00 | .35 | .49 | .60 | .69 | .77 |
| .80 | .00 | .40 | .57 | .69 | .80 | .89 |
| 1.00 | .00 | .45 | .63 | .77 | .89 | 1.00 |

Source: Adapted from Ghiselli and Brown, 1955.

of the predictor *or* the outcome measure is very low, it is impossible to have a predictive power high enough for any practical use. For example, assuming the true validity coefficient was 1.0 in the population, and given the reliability of the dependent measure was 0.80 and that of the independent measure only 0.40, then the highest possible validity coefficient for the independent variable as a predictor of the dependent variable would be 0.57. This is due to the unreliability of both measures. Table 9.4 does not show how high the validity coefficient will be when the reliability of both measures is known. Rather it shows the limits above which the validity cannot go. Even if the measures were perfectly reliable, the validity might still be zero. This last table illustrates how very important it is to achieve high levels of reliability in a measure. Thus, in cutting and pasting a new measure from an old one, item analyses and reliability assessment are of paramount importance.

## Procedures in the Construction of Factor-Analytic Measures

The purpose of using factor analysis in the development of measures is to determine the number of factors present in a set of items and to develop separate measures for each factor. Once the number of factors and the items defining each one have been determined, the procedure is exactly the same as was the case after item analysis. The only difference is the statistical criterion: The correlation of each item with the factor (factor loadings) should be greater than 0.3. All other criteria—length, content, percent of keyed response, computing Cronbach's alpha reliability and Ferguson's delta, and the subsequent item retrials—are the same as for item analysis.

The key asset of factor analysis is that it helps determine whether a set of items or parts of previous scales measure a single factor or more than one. If more than one factor is present in the data, an item analysis that assumes the items measure only one factor will be less successful. The presence of multiple factors in a set of items will result in a single measure having lower reliability than would be the case if separate factors were derived. Sample size is very important in producing stable factor solutions. It has been recommended by Nunnally (1978) that the ratio of subjects to items should be 10:1. Kline has shown, however, that a ratio of 3:1 gives results essentially identical to those with a ratio of 10:1. Kline (1986) further recommends a minimum sample size of 100 subjects even if relatively few items are tried out. This will help the researcher obtain replicable factors by reducing the standard errors of the correlations.

## Additional Psychometric Properties

Two additional aspects of the psychometric properties of scales deserve further emphasis. The first issue is that of norms. The norms include the scoring instructions, including weights and cutting scores if applicable, and the mean and standard deviation of the standardizing sample. They are used to compare an individual's score with the relevant normative group by means of some transformation that reveals that individual's status relative to the group. Standard scores are recommended, based on deviation of scores from the mean. Transformed standard scores are always comparable: the same standard scores being the same distance from the mean.

The second issue is that of replication or cross-validation on a new sample. Basing the results of an item analysis on a specific sample of persons tends to produce results that are less optimal when applied to new samples: Even with adequate sample size, shrinkage of correlations will occur. The effects are more pronounced when (a) the sample is small, (b) the number of items is large, and (c) the reliability is low. One strategy is to have a new or second sample and to repeat the item analysis on it. This procedure is called *cross-validation*. Formulas exist that estimate the amount of shrinkage expected based on the level of correlation, the number of items, and the sample size (Thorndike, 1982).

One of the difficulties faced in conducting cross-validation studies is the cost of such analyses. Constraints of resources often necessitate that the cross-validation be carried out as part of the original study. This means that the sample must be broken into two or more parts: a developmental sample and one or more cross-validation samples. Several strategies have been recommended for this. In the holdout group method, part of the sample is set aside as the cross-validation component; the remainder is used for the developmental phase. In the double cross-validation method, the available sample is split randomly in half and two separate developmental analyses are conducted; each is then cross-validated on the half of the original sample on which it was not developed. The final scale selection, especially if weights are involved, is often based on the combined data. Double cross-validation is strongly recommended as a more rigorous approach to the cross-validation of results from item analyses. Overall, cross-validation increases confidence in the resulting measure and provides a more realistic estimate of the performance of the measure in populations similar to the standardizing one.

## Factors Contributing to Low Reliability

Two situations can occur in which the resulting item analysis is unsuccessful, that is, the reliability of the final scale is too low to be of value. The first occurs when too many items are deleted from the original scale and new items are not written to take their place. In this situation not enough good items may be in the decimated item pool to produce a scale with adequate reliability. This inadequacy is always a danger when cutting and pasting new measures from old. The only recourse in this situation is to write additional items and to repeat the process of item analysis. A better strategy is to anticipate this possibility and include additional items from the original, if possible, or add new items from the onset.

A second situation contributing to poor scale reliability occurs when the item pool contains more than one factor or dimension. This is more likely to be a problem when new items are added to the item pool. Some of these items may measure factors that are not well correlated with the core dimension; such items will reduce the scale's reliability. One also runs the risk of mixing several factors when several scales purporting to measure the same construct are combined. If the factors correlate well, there is no problem. If they do not, however, and the investigators are unaware of the multiple factor structure of the different scales, then the reliability of the resulting composite measure may be significantly reduced. A factor analysis of the various scales prior to an attempt to combine them will help determine whether this situation is occurring in a given data set. One can then proceed to develop a composite measure based on the scales that measure a common concept.

## Precautions for Proceeding

The pitfalls are numerous in attempting to create new measures from old. First, many measures are copyrighted and require approval of the authors or the publishers. Still, many others that have been published are considered to be in the public domain. Measures are often published in journals or books to encourage investigators to use them in other contexts, thus adding to the empirical evidence of their construct validity. In the psychological field the Minnesota Multiphasic Personality Inventory is an example of a widely analyzed set of items with dozens of new scales developed from them.

A second pitfall concerns the need for adequate sample size to compute the required item and factor analyses. Without adequate sample size, biased item selection and capitalization on chance variations can substantially influence the results. Thus item selection and scale reliability are likely to include much random error variation. Such scales are less likely to replicate in the cross-validation analysis.

Another situation that frequently arises is the removal of an intact scale from a battery of scales. This situation gives rise to the possibility that items taken out of context may be responded to differently when imbedded among items from other scales than when they are administered together. An example of this would be if one selected, say, the anxiety scale from a measure comprised of a battery of scales. Would the scale perform as well in this context, and would the normative data from the battery be applicable to the isolated scale situation? The answers to those questions are not clear-cut except to emphasize that one should reevaluate scales administered in this way by using the procedures outlined in this chapter. Examining the items, the internal-consistency reliability, and the mean and standard deviation of the scale scores will provide ample evidence of the scale's performance in the new context. The current psychometric properties should be compared with those published for the scale when it was administered as part of a battery, to determine whether a consistent bias is present. The reliability may be the same, but the average scores may be consistently higher or lower. Having some estimate of the bias present is especially important in deciding what cutoff points to use in defining high-risk individuals. A cutoff point adjusted for such bias will enhance the scale's sensitivity and specificity when used in the new context.

Yet another pitfall involves the use of scales cross-culturally. Different ethnic groups may respond very differently to certain items or specific scale content. Language constraints often necessitate changes in item wording, content, or response style; scales that are to be used cross-culturally need to be translated and then back-translated to ensure consistency of meaning. Often new phrases need to be substituted for the original item content in order to achieve the same intent and meaning; simple word changes are often not adequate and may, on back translation, be found to distort seriously the original intent of the item. Thus extra effort is needed to prepare scales for cross-cultural use. This effort should include an evaluation of the psychometric properties of the items and the scale in the new cultural context. Such findings would be valuable in establishing the extent to which the scale's properties generalize to a new cultural setting, and it would also set up the opportunity to validate the construct cross-culturally.

The most straightforward application of these item analysis techniques is the situation in which one has taken a single old measure of a unidimensional construct and reduced it by deleting inappropriate items. The reasons for this may be a critical need to shorten the research protocol, or some items may simply be inappropriate or invalid for the population under study. Related to this reduction in item length is the situation in which new, more relevant items are written and included as part of the old abbreviated scale. The key issue here is the importance of knowing that one is dealing with an unidimensional scale. Although it is now modified from the original, the task is to reevaluate its psychometric properties and to determine whether it is reliable and valid for the purposes of the current study. The item analysis strategy described previously is the recommended way to proceed. Following these procedures will enable the researchers to determine whether the modified scale is a viable alternative to the original. Furthermore, documentation of the modified scale's item relationships, reliability, validity, and norms will allow other investigators to use it and to have greater confidence in its modified scores.

A situation that requires greater precaution and is more complex to evaluate is the one in which entire measures or selected items from two or more measures are combined to form a composite measure. Unless the measures are all of a single trait or attribute, the psychometric evaluation is considerably more complicated. In this situation a factor analysis of the item pool may be required to establish the number of different dimensions or factors present in the items. Next, separate item analyses would be conducted for each measurable factor. Finally, the methods of weighting and combining the factor scales into a composite measure require such advanced statistical techniques as second-order factor analysis or special regression techniques. The scoring, standardization, and norms for such measures are also more elaborate, often involving transformations of the composite scores. This situation calls for consultative input and help from a psychometrician or someone with expertise in these types of analyses.

## Summary

One of the reasons for placing such emphasis on item analysis is the need for brief measures in the clinical setting. Since many clinical encounters are only 10-15 minutes in length, it is imperative that assessments be brief in this context. This would make it practical to gather important data for research purposes within the context of a routine clinical visit. Otherwise, additional staff would be needed to administer the protocols, and patients would have to stay longer to complete the lengthier forms. Measures that are brief, reliable, and valid have many advantages. Such measures would enhance any clinical data base and allow a wide variety of clinical and epidemiological studies to be performed. Confidence in the use of brief measures, however, can come only from well-designed item and scale analyses. It is critical that their psychometric properties be well documented and cross-validated before they are placed in use in the clinical setting.

When cutting and pasting new measures from old, the process of evaluating the psychometric properties of the reconstituted measure is as important as when developing an original measure. In many ways the reconstituted measure is an unknown entity. One cannot assume a carryover effect of the original measure's psychometric properties. For longer measures with only a few items deleted, carryover effects might be expected to be high, but shorter measures with many items deleted would be expected to have fewer carryover effects. In a completely new population both might be expected to perform less well due to shrinkage and inappropriate items. As indicated above, a heavy emphasis is placed on maximizing the new scale's reliability. This is the key property for proceeding, since without adequate reliability the assessment of validity and the development of norms are unlikely to produce satisfactory results. Following the procedures outlined here will help ensure the construction of new or modified measures whose statistical, psychometric, and conceptual properties are more clearly understood.

## References

Allen, M. J., & Yen, W. M. (1979). *Introduction to measurement theory*. Belmont, CA: Wadsworth.

Bohrnstedt, G. W. (1969). A quick method for determining the reliability and validity of multiple-item scales. *American Sociological Review, 34,* 542-548.

Carmines, E. G., & Zeller, R. A. (1979). *Reliability and validity reassessment.* Beverly Hills, CA: Sage.

Edwards, A. L., (1970). *The measurement of personality traits by scales and inventories.* New York: Holt, Rinehart & Winston.

Ferguson, G. A. (1949). On the theory of test development. *Psychometrika, 14,* 61-68.

Ferguson, G. A. (1981). *Statistical analysis in psychology and education.* New York: McGraw-Hill.

Ghiselli, E. E., & Brown, C. W. (1955). *Personnel and Industrial Psychology.* New York: McGraw-Hill.

Gulliksen, H. (1950). *Theory of mental tests.* New York: John Wiley.

Guilford, J. P. (1954). *Psychometrics.* New York: McGraw-Hill.

Kline, P. (1986). *A handbook of test construction: Introduction to psychometric design.* London: Methuen.

Nie, N. H., Hull, C. H., Jenkins, J. G., Steinbrenner, K., & Bent, H. (Eds.). (1975). *Statistical package for the social sciences* (2nd ed.). New York: McGraw-Hill.

Nunnally, J. C. (1978). *Psychometric theory.* New York: McGraw-Hill.

Rust, J., & Golombok, S. (1982). *Modern psychometrics.* New York: Routledge.

Thorndike, R. L. (1982). *Applied psychometrics.* Boston: Houghton Mifflin.

# PART THREE

TOOLS FOR MEASUREMENT

# 10 Symptoms: Measures of the Mind

LARRY CULPEPPER

Primary care researchers frequently seek to measure symptoms. A symptom measure may be the independent variable, the outcome variable, or even both. For instance, the measurement of acute low back pain at first presentation may be of use in predicting chronic low back pain as an outcome. Symptoms also may be confounding variables.

To be useful in a research framework, symptoms must be measured by instruments that are known to be reliable and valid, as described in Chapters 5 and 6. Familiarity with these psychometric principles and instrument properties by themselves, however, is not sufficient to guide the researcher in selecting the best symptom scale for a particular study. To do this requires in addition an understanding of the neurophysiology underlying the symptom, the psychophysics involved in the perception and response to it, and the influence of the choice of scaling used in measurement. Also helpful is an appreciation of the nature of misclassification likely to occur with a particular instrument, and its impact on study results.

In this chapter the phenomenon of pain is used to illustrate concepts relevant to the selection of instruments for measuring symptoms as part of primary care research projects. Not covered is the much bigger task of developing new scales. This requires, in addition to mastery of the information in this chapter and in Chapter 6, skill in using the concepts developed in Chapter 8.

## Neurophysiology

The first step in choosing a symptom instrument is to review the basic neurophysiology underlying the symptom's perception. Of particular interest is identifying differences between closely related but distinct symptoms. For instance, if one is interested in a respiratory symptom such as dyspnea, an understanding of the difference in neurophysiologic mechanisms between pulmonary and cardiac sensations may be helpful. In the case of pain, insight is required into pain receptors, spinothalamic pathways, and cortical involvement in pain perception.

## Psychophysics

The primary care researcher will benefit from an understanding of psychophysics and its insights into the measurement of symptoms. A basic assumption underlying the measurement of symptoms is that the human experience of symptoms can be measured accurately. Psychophysics, which pertains to the way in which humans perceive and assess physical phenomena, provides evidence of the validity of this assumption (Gescheider, 1988).

Most people, when they look at two lines, one twice the length of the other, will accurately perceive this ratio relationship. Similarly, when given a number of pairs of sound stimuli, each pair including one sound twice the strength in decibels of the other, most people accurately perceive that the ratio relationship between the two sounds is constant across the different pairs. The doubling in sound intensity results in the same perceived intensity ratio whether the sound pairs are in the soft or very loud range. Instead of perceiving that the louder sound of each pair is twice the intensity of the softer, however, most people report it to be only two-thirds louder. Measurement of such perceptions is *psychophysics*. The basic research in psychophysics has led to findings that are relevant to the choice of scales for the measurement of pain and other sensory phenomena, particularly the comparison of magnitude and category scales.

While magnitude scales provide for a continuous response gradation and may be either ratio or absolute magnitude in nature, category scaling of symptom intensity yields ordinal level data (Young, 1984). For sensory phenomena (including pain) both types of scales can be shown to be reliable and valid (Anderson, 1970, 1976, 1982; Marks, 1974). When data produced by magnitude and category scales are compared, however, the relationship between the two types of scales is consistently nonlinear. At the low intensity range of the stimulus a greater degree of increase is reported using a category scale than a magnitude scale. Some have concluded that such nonlinearity is evidence that one or the other type of scale must be invalid.

When given an equally spaced set of categories to report the magnitude of a stimulus, subjects use increasing levels of the scale in a proportional rather than a linear manner (Lodge, 1981; Shinn, 1974). Thus small differences between low-intensity signals will be reported using different categories, while larger magnitude stimuli with the same absolute difference in intensity may be reported using the same category (Marks, 1968). For example, in reporting weights using a category scale, 6-oz and 2 lb-6 oz weights are apt to be judged as belonging to different categories (e.g., very light, and light), while 100-lb and 102-lb weights are judged to belong to the same category (very heavy). This results in a concave curvilinear relationship between category and magnitude estimation judgments, due to the nonlinear response to the category scale. Of note, nonlinearity has been shown to increase as the number of categories decreases. Therefore, if category scales are to be used in reporting symptom intensity, providing a large number of categories will minimize nonlinearity (Parducci & Wedell, 1986).

As already noted, one interpretation of the nonlinearity between magnitude and category scales has been that categorical scales must not be valid. An alternative explanation is that the two types of scales are measuring different aspects of perceptual experience and as such may be processed at different cognitive stages (Marks, 1979). While a continuous magnitude scale requires the reporting simply of sensation magnitude, category scales inevitably require the respondent to estimate sensory dissimilarity between the categories offered.

Thus the two types of scales may each have advantages. Magnitude scales may be best for measuring absolute magnitude, while category scales may be of use particularly in identifying the perception of differences. The primary care researcher should be aware of these issues and take them into account when choosing symptom measurement instruments.

## Instrument Selection

The selection of symptom measures for a research project should be based on a review of the literature. Three types of articles may be of value: reports of original research involving the symptom, research-oriented reviews regarding symptom measurement or relevant clinical conditions, and reports on individual symptom measurement tools. (For pain, the work of Deyo 1983; Greenland, Reisbord, Haldeman, & Buerger, 1980; Spitzer, LeBlanc, & Dupuis, 1986; and Waddell et al., 1982 are exemplary.)

The literature review is likely to identify a variety of instruments. The three issues already discussed should be considered for each. First, what is the theoretical basis, if any, for the instrument? (For example, for pain are the underlying neurophysiologic, psychologic, or social dimensions incorporated into the theoretical framework of the instrument?) Second, do concepts of psychophysics support the measurement approach used by the instrument? Third, what are the psychometric properties (reliability and validity) of the instrument (Wittenborn, 1972)?

The final selection of an instrument should be based on a number of additional criteria:

1. Does the instrument's content fit the purpose of the study?
2. Is the measure too narrow or too broad?
3. Is the level of scale discrimination right?
4. Is the ability to measure change adequate?
5. If multidimensional, are individual scale items and weights appropriate for the study?
6. Is the reading level appropriate for study subjects, and is the measure culturally appropriate?
7. Is the respondent burden too great?

These seven issues are part of the consideration of a basic trade-off of cost versus information yield. The efforts of administration, scoring and entering data, and the complexity of analysis are all "costs." Another aspect of this trade-off is the completeness and accuracy of information versus the amount of information. Simple, brief instruments are likely to result in a higher rate of completion and a lower rate of nonresponse but less information than more complex instruments. Substantial nonresponse will affect the power of the study and increase the number of subjects needed, and it also may affect study validity.

## Measurement Tools Available to Assess Symptoms

A number of approaches may be used to measure symptoms. While self-report has been the mainstay of symptom measurement, the incorporation of an objective behavioral tool (such as a pain medication pill-count) may provide an easily understood complementary measure.

Of limited use in primary care are the laboratory techniques used in the basic research of the psychophysics of sensations. The addition of laboratory standardization or concurrent validation of study instruments using a small subset of subjects and traditional laboratory psychophysical techniques may be of interest.

Observational techniques generally report behaviors of patients. Such behaviors may be voluntary or involuntary, such as limping, coughing, restricted range of motion, or grimacing. Generally, observational techniques should be as unobtrusive as possible. Alternatively, subjects may be asked to perform a set routine of activities while being observed in a standardized manner. (Waddell, McCulloch, Kummel, & Venner [1980] and Craig & Prkachin [1983] have discussed observational approaches to pain measurement, and Fordyce [1976] has reviewed the relationship between overt pain behavior and self-report.)

Assessment of utilization is a specific type of observational technique. Use of medication, use of health services, and use of sick days are all possible surrogate measures for symptom intensity. For example, pain medication use and days off work may be appropriate measures for the assessment of low back pain. Each is subject to its own set of confounders, and the measurement of such may greatly improve a study. Behavioral measures may be of particular value when the research is planned with relevance to public policy in mind. Such measures have the advantage of being easily understood by nonclinical policymakers.

Functional assessment may be used as an indirect measure of symptoms. Functional ability may be either observed or self-reported. Particularly for pain this approach is frequently used. For acute pain it may be correlated closely with pain intensity or other pain qualities. For chronic pain the psychological and social dimensions of pain may be the dominant factors related to functional performance. The Oswestry Low Back Pain Disability Questionnaire is a good example of a symptom-related function scale (Fairbank, Couper, Davies, & O'Brien, 1980).

Self-report measures are the most frequently used approaches to symptom measurement. These generally are questionnaires, although for some studies a diary approach may be of value.

McDowell and Newell (1987) provide an overview of eight pain-related instruments, most of which are questionnaires. This reference also reviews instruments for many other dimensions of health and should be part of any primary care research library.

Qualitative approaches should be considered seriously in assessing symptoms. Such approaches as the Long Interview or focus groups may be of particular value in exploring the dimensions of a symptom. This exploration may be very helpful in the early stages of a research effort and may provide insights that help guide the selection of quantitative study instruments. (See Chapters 15 and 16.)

## Examples of Instruments

This section describes three examples of pain measurement instruments: the visual analog scale, the McGill Pain Questionnaire, and pain drawings.

### VISUAL ANALOG PAIN SCALES

The visual analog scale (VAS) is basically a straight line that represents the symptom range to be rated (Huskisson, 1974, 1982; Scott & Huskisson, 1976). For pain, one end of the scale is labelled *no pain,* and the other end *pain as bad as it could be.* The respondent is asked to mark the line at a point corresponding to the severity of the pain. This technique generally takes about 30 seconds and provides a simple summary measure of pain intensity. Instructions should define whether the pain is as experienced now, in the last 24 hours, in the last week, or some other interval, and whether the most intense or average pain is to be reported.

McDowell and Newell (1987) discuss visual analog scales and cite studies of their psychometric properties. Different line lengths, vertical and horizontal line placement, and defining only the two ends or in addition points along the line have all been evaluated (See also Revill, Robinson, Rosen, & Hogg [1976]; and Scott & Huskisson [1979]). Based on these assessments the line should be at least 10 cm long and, unless the respondent population can be predicted to have trouble with the measure otherwise, should not have labels along its length. Vertical or horizontal lines yield equally good results.

About 7% of people asked to use a VAS cannot do so because of confusion in understanding the underlying concepts (Huskisson, 1974). The use of a numerical rating scale (i.e., "rate your pain from 1 to 100") can be used by all but 1-2% of most populations. Numerical rating and visual analog techniques have been combined in the development of a line with numbers attached (Downie et al., 1978). As with categorical scales a larger number of labeled points may improve scale performance. Generally a reasonable compromise may be the visual analog line-length approach modified to have 10 equally spaced numbers along its length.

Scoring of a VAS may be based on the actual distance of the respondent's mark from the lower end of the scale. Alternatively a 20-point grid may be superimposed on the line to give a categorical rating; this approach represents the maximum level of discrimination used by most in recording pain levels (Huskisson, 1974). Scoring procedures have been reviewed critically by Maxwell (1978). The distribution of results is not normal, so transformations of scores or nonparametric analytic techniques may be appropriate (Huskisson, 1982; Maxwell, 1978).

A related issue is the use of a VAS at multiple points in time to identify symptom change. One view is that such use is fundamentally inappropriate (Dixon & Bird, 1981; Huskisson, 1974) since the initial measurement point bounds the range of change possible in a decidedly nonnormal manner. For instance, if the initial rating of pain is 8 on a 10-cm scale, the respondent is limited to a 2-cm range to describe all degrees of worsening pain but has an 8-cm range to describe pain improvement on subsequent reports. Other approaches that have been proposed include using a VAS with the endpoints of *no relief* to *complete relief* of pain. Alteratively the midpoint could be *no relief,* with one endpoint being *complete relief* and the other endpoint being *severe worsening* of the pain. Both of these approaches may be difficult for subjects to understand. Therefore neither the repeat use of the VAS nor the use of a "pain change" VAS may perform well. To assess change in pain intensity, a simple descriptive categorical scale may give better results.

## The McGill Pain Questionnaire

This questionnaire has been the standard of the field and has had its reliability and validity assessed for numerous populations (Melzack, 1975). It is based on a theoretical conceptualization of pain as having three distinct dimensions: sensory-discriminative, motivational-affective, and cognitive-evaluative. Melzack (1973), in constructing this instrument, theorized that these three dimensions are served by distinct neurologic systems.

Twenty groups of two to six words are presented, and respondents are asked to select a word in each group if it describes their pain. No word is chosen if none in the group apply. Through a series of studies with students, physicians, and patients, scale weights were determined for each word within each category and a scoring system validated. Included are a 5-point categorical pain intensity scale, simple pain drawing, and categorical scales that describe accompanying symptoms, effects on sleep, effects on food intake, and activity level. The instrument takes about 5 minutes to complete.

The instrument may be used to describe average pain, most intense pain, typical pain, pain now, or other pain conceptualizations and has been used to assess both acute and chronic pain. It has been translated and revalidated in several languages; also some investigators in other countries have used the same developmental procedures to create analogous questionnaires (DeBenedittis, Massei, Nobili, & Pieri, 1988; Pöntinen & Ketovuori, 1983). (The report of the development of the Italian Pain Questionnaire by DeBenedittis and his colleagues provides a particularly elegant description of this.)

Varying but generally similar results have been obtained by different investigators conducting factor analyses using different populations (Crocket, Prkachin, & Craig, 1977; Prieto & Geisinger, 1983; Prieto et al., 1980; Reading, 1979). McDowell and Newell (1987) note a number of conceptual difficulties in using factor analysis to assess the validity of the questionnaire. These include the fact that the correlation of words in any one group must be zero since respondents select only one word per group. Thus the qualitative homogeneity of words in the groups cannot be tested empirically. Another concern is that pain quality and intensity are measured concurrently by the use of the words, and these dimensions may be mixed in the factor analysis reporting (Leavitt, Garron, Whisler, & Sheinkop, 1978; Melzack & Torgerson, 1971).

## The Pain Drawing

A number of investigators have used a pain drawing instrument (Hildebrandt, Franz, Choroba-Mehnen, & Temme, 1988; Udén, Åström & Bergenudd, 1988) in which the respondent is given a line drawing of a human torso and asked to shade in the areas corresponding to the distribution of his or her pain. Various cross-hatchings can be used to enable reporting the localization of pain, intensity gradations, and pain qualities.

The pain drawing originally was conceived to identify pain magnification or nonanatomical pain distribution. This use was proposed as a means of differentiating nonorganic chronic low back pain patients from those with organic causes (Murphy & Cornish, 1984; Taylor, Stern, & Kubiszyn, 1984). While early reports were promising, later reports have shown the instrument to perform only moderately well for this purpose (Dennis, Rocchio, & Wiltse, 1981; Dzoiba, & Doxey, 1984; Leavitt, 1982; Margolis, Chibnall, & Tait, 1988; Schwartz & De Good, 1984; Udén et al., 1988). The correlation is poor also between pain drawings and specific psychological attributes (Hildebrandt et al., 1988; von Baeyer, Bergstrom, Brodwin, & Brodwin, 1983). The Ransford Scoring System was developed to differentiate organic and nonorganic pain; elements of it may be useful to the primary care investigator (Ransford, Cairns, & Mooney, 1976).

While the pain drawing has not been validated for the original purpose proposed, it still may be a valuable technique for primary care researchers. It may provide insight into pain (or other symptoms) and may be helpful particularly in exploratory studies. It may be considered a qualitative technique and may be combined with other qualitative approaches such as the Long Interview. The development of quantitative scaling methods for primary care research purposes still needs investigation.

## Conclusion

The choice of measurement instruments for a research project, along with careful development of inclusion and exclusion criteria and sample size determination, are fundamental to the validity of any research endeavour. Whenever possible, preexisting instruments should be chosen rather than the creation of new sets of questions or other measures. The selection of an instrument should be based on an understanding of the fundamental biological properties underlying the symptom, the psychophysics involved in symptom perception and reporting, the psychometric properties of the instruments available, and the applicability and usefulness of the instrument for the specific research project. For most instruments a body of literature exists that can help guide evaluation. Instrument choice usually depends on a trade-off between the financial and nonfinancial costs related to the instrument and the information that it will yield.

## References

Anderson, N. H. (1970). Functional measurement and psychophysical judgment. *Psychological Review, 77*, 153-170.

Anderson, N. H. (1976). Integration theory, functional measurement, and the psychological law. In H. G. Geisslerl & Y. M. Zabrodin (Eds.), *Advances in psychophysics* (pp. 99-130). Berlin: VEB Deutscher Verlag.

Anderson, N. H. (1982). Cognitive algebra and social psychophysics. In B. Wegener (Ed.). *Social attitudes and psychophysical measurement* (pp. 123-148). Hillsdale, NJ: Lawrence Erlbaum.

Craig, K. D., & Prkachin, K. M. (1983). Nonverbal measures of pain. In R. Melzack (Ed.), *Pain measurement and assessment* (pp. 173-179). New York: Raven Press.

Crockett, D. J., Prkachin, K. M., & Craig, K. D. (1977). Factors of the language of pain in patient and volunteer groups. *Pain, 4*, 175-182.

DeBenedittis, G., Massei, R., Nobili, R., & Pieri, A. (1988). The Italian Pain Questionnaire. *Pain, 33*, 53-62.

Dennis, M. D., Rocchio, P. O., & Wiltse, L. L. (1981). The topographical pain representation and its correlation with MMPI scores. *Orthopedics, 5*(4), 432-434.

Deyo, R. A., & Centor, R. M. (1986). Assessing the responsiveness of functional scales to clinical change: An analogy to diagnostic test performance. *Journal of Chronic Diseases, 39*(11), 897-906.

Deyo, R. A. (1983). Conservative therapy for low back pain; Distinguishing useful from useless therapy. *Journal of the American Medical Association, 250,* 1057-1062.

Dixon, J. S., & Bird, H. A. (1981). Reproducibility along a 10 cm vertical visual analogue scale. *Annals of the Rheumatic Diseases, 40,* 87-89.

Downie, W. W., Leatham, P. A., Rhind, V. M., Wright, V., Branco, J. A., & Anderson, J. A. (1978). Studies with pain rating scales. *Annals of the Rheumatic Diseases, 37,* 378-381.

Duda, P. D. (1967). Effects of procedural differences in ratio scaling techniques. *Canadian Psychologist, 8,* 161.

Dzioba, R. B., & Doxey, N. C. (1984). A prospective investigation into the orthopaedic and psychologic predictors of outcome of first lumbar surgery following industrial injury. *Spine, 9,* 614-623.

Fairbank, J. C. T., Couper, J., Davies, J. B., & O'Brien, J. P. (1980). The Oswestry low back pain disability questionnaire. *Physiotherapy, 66,* 271-273.

Fordyce, W. E. (1976). *Behavioral methods for chronic pain and illness.* St. Louis: C. V. Mosby.

Gescheider, G. A. (1988). Psychophysical scaling. *Annual Review of Psychology, 39,* 169-200.

Greenland, S., Reisbord, R. P. T., Haldeman, D. C., & Buerger, A. A. (1980). Controlled clinical trials of manipulation: A review and proposal. *Journal of Occupational Medicine, 22,* 670-676.

Hildebrandt, J., Franz, C. E., Choroba-Mehnen, B., & Temme, M. (1988). The use of pain drawings in screening for psychological involvement in complaints of low-back pain. *Spine, 13*(6), 681-685.

Huskisson, E. C. (1974). Measurement of pain. *Lancet, 2,* 1127-1131.

Huskisson, E. C. (1982). Measurement of pain. *Journal of Rheumatology, 9,* 768-769.

Leavitt, F. (1982). Comparison of three measures for detecting psychological disturbance in patients with low back pain. *Pain, 13,* 299-305.

Leavitt, F., Garron, D. C., Whisler, W. W., & Sheinkop, M. B. (1978). Affective and sensory dimensions of back pain. *Pain, 4,* 273-281.

Lodge, M. (1981). *Magnitude scaling: Quantitative measurement of opinions.* Beverly Hills, CA: Sage. (Sage University Papers, Series on Quantitative Applications in the Social Sciences, No. 07-001.)

Margolis, R. B., Chibnall, J. T., & Tait, R. C. (1988). Test-retest reliability of the pain drawing instrument. *Pain, 33,* 49-51.

Marks, L. E. (1968). Stimulus-range, number of categories, and form of the category scale. *American Journal of Psychology, 81,* 467-479.

Marks, L. E. (1974). On scales of sensation: Prolegomena to any future psychophysics that will come forth as science. *Perception and Psychophysics, 16,* 358-376.

Marks, L. E. (1979). A theory of loudness and loudness judgments. *Psychology Review, 86,* 256-285.

Maxwell, C. (1978). Sensitivity and accuracy of the visual analogue scale: A psychophysical classroom experiment. *British Journal of Pharmacology, 6,* 15-24.

McDowell, I., Newell, C. (1987). *Measuring health: A guide to rating, scales and questionnaires.* New York: Oxford University Press.

Melzack, R. (1973). *The puzzle of pain.* New York: Basic Books.

Melzack, R. (1975). The McGill Pain Questionnaire: Major properties and scoring methods. *Pain, 1,* 277-299.

Melzack, R., & Torgerson, W. S. (1971). On the language of pain. *Anesthesiology, 34,* 50-59.

Murphy, K. A., Cornish, R. D. (1984). Prediction of chronicity in acute low back pain. *Archives of Physiological and Medical Rehabilitation, 65,* 334-337.

Parducci, A., & Wedell, D. (1986). The category effect with rating scales: number of categories, number of stimuli, and method of presentation. *Journal of Experiments in Psychology, Human Perception and Performance, 12,* 496-516.

Pöntinen, P. J., & Ketovuori, H. (1983). Verbal measurement in non-English language: The Finnish Pain Questionnaire. In R. Melzack (Ed.), *Pain measurement and assessment* (pp. 85-93). New York: Raven Press.

Prieto, E. J., & Geisinger, K. F. (1983). Factor-analytic studies of the McGill Pain Questionnaire. In R. Melzack (Ed.), *Pain measurement and assessment* (pp. 63-70). New York: Raven Press.

Prieto, E. J., Hopson, L., Bradley, L. A., Byrne, M., Geisinger, K. F., Midax, D., & Marchisello, P. J. (1980). The language of low back pain: Factor structure of the McGill Pain Questionnaire. *Pain, 8,* 11-19.

Ransford, A. O., Cairns, D., & Mooney, V. (1976). The pain drawing as an aid to the psychologic evaluation of patients with low-back pain. *Spine, 1,* 127-134.

Reading, A. E. (1979). The internal structure of the McGill Pain Questionnaire in dysmenorrhoea patients. *Pain, 7,* 353-358.

Revill, S. I., Robinson, J. O., Rosen, M., & Hogg, M. I. J. (1976). The reliability of a linear analogue for evaluating pain. *Anaesthesia, 31,* 1191-1198.

Schwartz, D. P., & De Good, D. E. (1984). Global appropriateness of pain drawings: Blind ratings predict patterns of psychological distress and ligitation status. *Pain, 19,* 383-388.

Scott, J., & Huskisson, E. C. (1976). Graphic representation of pain. *Pain, 2,* 175-184.

Scott, J., & Huskisson, E. C. (1979). Vertical or horizontal visual analogue scales. *Annals of the Rheumatic Diseases, 38,* 560.

Shinn, A. M., Jr. (1974). Relations between scales. In H. M. Blalock, Jr. (Ed.), *Measurement in the social sciences: Theories and strategies.* Chicago: Aldine.

Spitzer, W. O., LeBlanc, F. E., & Dupuis, M. (1986). Scientific approach to the assessment and management of activity-related spinal disorders [Special supplement]. Commissioned and funded by the Institute for Workers' Health and Safety of Quebec (Institute de la recherche en sante et en Securite au travail), *Spine,* February.

Taylor, W. P., Stern, V. R., & Kubiszyn, T. W. (1984). Predicting patients' perceptions of response to treatment for low-back pain. *Spine, 9,* 313-316.

Udén, A., Åström, M., & Bergenudd, H. (1988). Pain drawings in chronic back pain. *Spine, 13*(4), 389-392.

von Baeyer, C. L., Bergstrom, K. J., Brodwin, M. G., & Brodwin, S. K. (1983). Invalid use of pain drawings in psychological screening of back pain patients. *Pain, 16,* 103-107.

Waddell, G., Main, C. J., Morris, E. W., Venner, R. M., Rae, P. S., Sharmy, S. H., & Galloway, H. (1982). Normality and reliability in the clinical assessment of backache. *British Medical Journal [Clinical Research], 284,* 1519-1523.

Waddell, G., McColloch, J., Kummel, E., & Venner, R. (1980). Nonorganic physical signs in low back pain. *Spine, 5,* 117-125.

Wittenborn, J. R. (1972). Reliability, validity, and objectivity of symptom-rating scales. *Journal of Nervous and Mental Disorders, 154,* 79-87.

Young, F. W. (1984). Scaling. *Annual Review of Psychology, 35,* 55-81.

# 11  Quality of Life and the Assessment of Primary Care

## J. IVAN WILLIAMS

The goals of health care include the maintenance of health, the prevention of disease, the treatment of disease, the management of chronic and disabling conditions, and palliative care. What health care seeks to avoid can be expressed in terms of the seven Ds: **D**eath, **D**isability, **D**isruption, **D**iscomfort, **D**isease, **D**issatisfaction, and **D**estitution—that is, the negative impact of the effects of disease and its management. In this context *health* is defined as "the absence of negative events."

Working from the World Health Organization's definition of *health* as "physical, social, and emotional well-being," researchers have sought to express the impact of health care in positive terms. This concept of health status includes five distinct components: physical health, mental health, social functioning, role functioning, and general health perceptions; some experts would add pain as a sixth component. During the 1970s teams of investigators developed measures of health status. These include the Health Status Measures developed by the Rand group for the Health Insurance Experiment (Brook et al., 1983), the McMaster Health Questionnaire Index (Chambers, 1988), the Nottingham Health Profile (Hunt, McEwen, & McKenna, 1985), the Sickness Impact Profile (Bergner, Bobbit, Carter, & Gilson, 1981), and the Index of Well-Being and the Quality of Well-Being Index (Kaplan & Bush, 1982) developed by the San Diego group. More recently Stewart, Hays, and Ware (1988) developed a short form of the Rand measures for use in the Major Outcomes Study. These and other measures are multidimensional and include all or most of the components outlined above. Health status influences the quality of life, but it does not determine it. Quality of life includes other components as well, and the use and comprehensiveness of the term varies from writer to writer.

The term *quality* has the same meaning as *grade* or *rank*, which can range from high to low or best to worst. Countries can be ranked on their economies and on the types and amounts spent by governments on social programs relative to expenditures on the military and industry. At the individual level the indicators of interest can be objective (for example, job, income, shelter, food, appliances) or subjective (happiness, sense of well-being, self-realization, perceptions of worth, value of life).

The best known studies of the quality of life of individuals are those of Andrews and Withey (1976) and Campbell (Campbell, 1981; Campbell, Converse, & Rodgers, 1976) at the Institute for Social Research at the University of Michigan. Both teams of investigators asked questions about multiple facets of life satisfaction, including work, marriage, health, leisure activities, family, housing, and neighborhood. They developed a global measure of satisfaction by combining the ratings across the items.

Quality-of-life studies in the health sector are more limited in scope. In health care the task at hand is to assess the impact of disease and interventions on the well-being of the patient. The patient's perception of the resulting health status may influence his or her sense of life satisfaction but not determine it. As Ware (1987) has noted, "jobs, housing, schools, and the neighborhood are not attributes of an individual's health, and they are well outside the purview of the health care system" (Ware, 1987, p. 474). The purpose of this chapter is to provide an overview of how the concept of quality-of-life has been developed and applied in research and to explore various approaches and measures used in health care research.

## Traditional Endpoints in Health Care

Fletcher, Fletcher, and Wagner (1988) list the following traditional clinical endpoints of health care: survival, evidence of improvement, remission of symptoms, and recurrence of disease. These indicators are used in quality-of-life studies, particularly when the diseases or conditions are life-threatening.

Symptom checklists and visual analog scales are direct and simple methods to measure clinical endpoints. Patients can check their ratings quickly on visual analog scales, linear analog self-assessment scales, Likert scales, or other categories for recording responses. The major problem is that the list of symptoms varies from condition to condition and from one treatment to another. The checklists tend not to be standardized, and minimal attention is paid to the reliability and validity of the scores. Checklists and linear analog scales have become the "quick and dirty" measures of quality of care. They provide more information than traditional clinical endpoints. In fact they provide relatively useful information about the impact of the disease and its management on the well-being of the patients.

## Indices of Functional Disability and Health Status Measures

Disability is a major component of the burden of ill health (Haynes, 1988). Feinstein, Josephy, and Wells (1986) reviewed the literature and found 43 widely used indices that focus in whole or in part on activities of daily living. Neither the reliability nor validity have been established for most of these measures.

The Sickness Impact Profile, the Rand health status measures, and the Nottingham Health Profile are used fairly routinely in assessments of health care, particularly with ambulatory patients in the community. These instruments are multidimensional, and investigators are reluctant to use them intact either because of length or because of lack of items apparently sensitive to the problem or intervention under study. Sometimes investigators have either used part of health status measures or added and deleted items.

The Duke-UNC Health Profile (Parkerson et al., 1981) is one measure that has been developed specifically for use in family practice. Parkerson and colleagues (1989) also have developed the Duke Social Support and Distress Scale to measure social functioning. To date, neither instrument has been compared with the measures noted above.

It can be noted that the physical functioning components of the various measures are similar in content, and they are reasonably comparable. In contrast the components for psychological functioning, role performance, and social functioning vary more dramatically from one instrument to another.

The social dimensions of health—social functioning and social support—have proven particularly difficult to assess. No single measure works as well for these as do the various measures for physical and psychological dimensions. Ware (1987) believes that the dimension of social functioning is sufficiently distant in concept from health and disease that it should be dropped from measures of health status and quality of life.

## Disease-Specific Quality-of-Life Measures

Some researchers argue that quality-of-life measures should be disease-specific in order to detect important clinical changes when assessing interventions (Guyatt, Bombardier, & Tugwell, 1986). For example, Levine and his colleagues (1988), when developing the Breast Cancer Questionnaire, decided to construct an instrument that would be disease-specific while addressing physical, emotional, and social well-being. They reported that the instrument was sensitive to important changes in therapy, but quality-of-life and functional status measures were not. Other notable quality-of-life measures that are cancer-specific include Padilla's Quality of Life Index (Padilla & Grant, 1985; Padilla et al., 1983), Karnofsky's Index of Performance Status (Karnofsky & Burchemal, 1949), and Schipper's Functional Living Index—Cancer (Schipper, Clinch, McMurray, & Levitt, 1984). Guyatt and his colleagues (1986) have worked to develop quality-of-life measures for other conditions and problems as well.

Disease-specific measures are limited in scope and focus, and the results from studies of various interventions and diseases are generally not comparable. These measures, however, are important to include in randomized clinical trials when the targeted outcomes go beyond clinical endpoints to include functioning, affect, and psychological well-being.

## Measures of Psychological Well-Being

Some researchers have turned to measures of psychological well-being, mood, and affect as indicators of quality of life. Hollandsworth (1988) reviewed quality-of-life studies published from 1980 through 1984, as an update of a 5-year review article (1975-1979) by Najman and Levine (1981). The Affect Balance Scale (Bradburn, 1969), the Health Locus of Control Scale (Wallston, Kaplan, & Maides, 1976), the Profile of Mood States (McNair, Lorr, & Drappleman, 1971), and Rosenberg's Self-Esteem Scale (Rosenberg, 1962) are among the psychological measures that have been used as indicators of quality of life in medical care studies. Dupuy (1973) developed the General Well-Being Schedule for use in the United States National Health Survey. Ware and his associates (1984) adapted it to create the Mental Health Inventory for use in the Rand Health Insurance Experiment.

The measures mentioned above focus on the positive features of emotional well-being. Symptom checklists for psychological and psychiatric problems may be used as well. The investigator may choose to use standardized psychological checklists in addition to or in place of health status measures with psychological dimensions. The standard scores obtained from the checklists come at the expense of length due to the added items.

## Quality of Life and Life Satisfaction Measures

In a review of measures for the Institute of Medicine Council on Health Care Technology, Williams and Wood-Dauphinee (1989) identified three global measures of quality of life related to health care. The best known measure is the Quality-of-Life Index developed by Spitzer and his colleagues (1981). It has five dimensions: principal activity, activities of daily living, perception of health, social support, and outlook on life. The responses indicate whether the patient is compromised, limited, or unlimited in each area by health problems. The total score ranges between 0 and 10. Chubon (1985, 1986, 1987) and Ferrans and Powers (1985) each developed multidimensional measures that would be applicable for both healthy individuals and for patients ill with a variety of problems. These measures, however, have not been used widely.

Life satisfaction measures may serve as global indicators of quality of life in health care. Measures developed at the University of Michigan have been adapted for studies in the health care field (Andrews & Withey, 1976; Campbell, 1981). Neugarten, Havighurst, and Tobin (1961) have created life satisfaction measures for their studies of the aged, and the Philadelphia Geriatric Center Morale Scale was developed by Lawton (1975) for the same purpose.

## Utility Assessments of Quality of Life

The measures for quality of life discussed thus far provide a rating or ranking of the health state of the individual. Such ratings, however, do not indicate what the value or worth of that health state is to the individual or to society at large. Utility assessments are designed to address these questions. They have two components: the judgment of the value or worth of life at a given point in time, and the quantity or years of life spent in a given health state.

The utility assessments have been derived from a theoretical perspective and methodology distinct from those employed by behavioral and clinical scientists. The general approach is based on modern utility theory as advanced by von Neumann and Morgenstern (1953). Major groups of researchers responsible for applying utility theory to the health care field include the late James Bush, Robert Kaplan, and their colleagues at the University of California at San Diego; Rachel Rosser and her colleagues at Charing Cross Hospital in London; George Torrance and his colleagues at McMaster University in Hamilton, Ontario; and Milton Weinstein and his colleagues (1980) at Harvard University. Torrance (1986, 1987); Anderson, Bush, and Berry (1988); and Kaplan and his associates (Kaplan, Atkins, & Times, 1984; Kaplan & Bush, 1982) have published information on the reliability and validity of their methods.

The McMaster group has used three approaches in deriving the utility values: the standard gamble technique, the time trade-off method, and rating scales. The standard gamble technique, the original method, is based directly on the axioms of utility theory. Here the subject uses the standard gamble to choose between two alternatives to treatment. Let us suppose that the outcome for a new surgical technique leads to a 70% chance of restoration to normal health but a 30% chance exists of permanent disability or death. The usual surgical procedures nearly always lead to some reduction in the capacity in functional status, say 25% of normal, but rarely result in death or disability. The probabilities associated with the new outcome ($p$ for normal life, $1-p$ for death or disability) can be varied until the individual expresses no real difference in choice between the interventions. The utility value is the probability of achieving normal health with the new surgical technique ($p = 0.70$).

Torrance, Thomas, and Sackett (1972) developed the time trade-off method as an alternative that is simpler to apply. The individual is asked to consider a health state, say relatively stable angina, that is to last for a fixed period of time, say 10 years. A new procedure will give the individual normal health for a shorter time period, for example 7 years, but the individual will probably die or be severely disabled at that time. The individual is asked to "trade off" the time with reduced capacity for living with lesser time in normal health. The time in normal health is varied until the point of indifference is found. The utility value is derived by dividing the time in normal health by the time with reduced capacity ($p = 0.70 = 7/10$).

In developing the rating scale approach, Torrance, Boyle, and Horwood (1982) specified six attributes that should be included in a health state: physical function, emotional function, sensory function, cognitive function, self-care, and pain. Each attribute is given several levels of gradation, and the characteristics of a given health state would include a description of the levels of functioning, self-care, and pain associated with the attributes that are associated with that state. The above descriptions of hypothetical persons in various health states can be narrated in written vignettes, videotapes, or in other forms. The ratings assigned to the descriptions are placed on a visual analog scale ranging from 0 to 100. Multiple Attribute Theory is used to determine the value for each level of each attribute and the utility value of the particular combinations of attributes found in a given health state. Torrance (1987) presented a summary of the reliability ratings and tests of validity for the utility values derived by the above three methods.

These methods do have problems: They are time-consuming, demanding of subjects, require skilled interviewers, and are costly to apply. They have been modified to simplify the tasks, and the McMaster group reports participation and completion rates of at least 85%.

The San Diego group took a different approach to assessing utility values (Kaplan et al., 1984; Kaplan & Bush, 1982). Their first step was to place individuals with given health states into categories of mobility, physical activity, and social activity. The second step was to classify the symptoms and health problems that these individuals have on a given day. Then 400 case descriptions were written to encompass the combinations of functional levels and symptoms or problems.

Random samples of individuals in the community gave preference ratings for the descriptions. Weights were derived for each level of mobility, physical activity, social activity, and symptom or problem. Quality of Well-Being (QWB) scores were computed by combining the weights into utility values for the health states. In a study comparing the reliability of assessments obtained by personal interviews and self-administered forms, Anderson, Bush, and Berry (1988) concluded that personal interviews are required for reliable QWB scores.

Several difficulties remain. Should utility values be obtained from the public at large, the providers of health care, and the patients themselves, or should they reflect the assessments of the family members whose lives are directly affected by the quality of life of the patients? Debate continues about whether a proxy rating by a significant other should be obtained for patients who are unable to form judgments for themselves. Patients' assessments of their health states change as their conditions change; consequently the utility values may not be stable over time. Assumptions about morbidity, disability, prognosis, and life expectancy are based on expert opinion, as sound epidemiological data on the natural history of disease and the effects of interventions are generally not available. Finally, while agreement may exist that utility values provide a ranking of conditions, far less agreement exists about whether they can be equated with judgments about the worth of lives of persons who are in these health states.

## Choices and Decisions About Quality of Life Measures

Given the lack of agreement about what is meant by quality of life, I am not surprised that it is assessed with a plethora of measures and research strategies. The choices reflect the professional training of the investigators and their preference for strategies. As it may be difficult to find measures that appear to address particular clinical problems completely, it is understandable that investigators are inclined to create their own measures. These created measures increases the diversity of instruments and approaches in assessing quality of life.

Given the abundance of measures that have been created or transposed from the behavioral and social sciences, no clear-cut choices exist about the instruments that should be used in a given study. Some guidelines and criteria do exist, however, for making choices and rules, and some tools can be employed in assessing the reliability and validity of particular measures. One general rule of thumb is that an investigator should not set out to create a new measure unless convinced that available instruments fail to meet the requirements of the intended study.

## Thinking About the Content

The validity of the content of a measure is frequently taken for granted. If measures or items seem to be related to the health problem or intervention, it is assumed that the items have face or content validity. Yet several issues have to be addressed implicitly or explicitly in the selection of measures or items. The first has been addressed already: The selections can be disease-specific or applicable to a range of problems and interventions. Second, they may focus on either traditional clinical endpoints, the outcomes that are assessed near the time of diagnosis and treatment, or on long-range outcomes. Third, a choice exists between measuring objective and subjective variables. Objective measures are based on variables that can be observed independently of the subject and recorded by various testing procedures and observations by assessors.

Measures of disease activity, remission of symptoms, presence of side effects, changes in functional capacity, ability to carry out usual activities, and family and social activities are phenomena that can be observed and recorded by someone other than the subject. Subjective measures, in contrast, provide opportunities for individuals to express their own thoughts, knowledge, attitudes, motivations, moods, and feelings. In the case of quality of life, investigators generally prefer that patients rate their own. Proxy assessments may be possible if patients are unable to respond for themselves.

Timing of the assessments is important. Measures such as the linear analog, self-assessment scales, the Functional Living Index—Cancer, and the Breast Cancer Questionnaire are designed for repeated use before, during, and immediately after treatment to assess patients' short-term responses during the course of therapy. Such global measures as the Spitzer Quality-of-Life Index are designed to reflect the quality of life remaining following the treatment of disease. Coates et al. (1987) and Levine et al. (1988) have used the Spitzer Quality-of-Life Index short-term assessment during a trial, but the scores tend to be less responsive to clinical changes than the disease-specific measures.

It should be noted that a particular problem exists with repeated self-assessments during the course of therapy. Investigators have found it difficult to maintain high completion rates over the testings (Finkelstein et al., 1988; Raghavan, Grundy, & Lancaster, 1988), and their use of the data was limited by the missing values. Levine et al. (1988) minimized the loss of data by having nurses interview the patients during clinic visits, but this procedure adds significantly to the time and costs of the study.

It is not uncommon for investigators simply to choose those items and measures they feel to be most directly relevant for their study. The most complete approach would include a systematic review of the literature, consultations with health professionals who share the responsibilities, and discussions with the patients and their significant others. An additional step is to have all interested parties, particularly patients and those close to them, rank the measures or items in terms of prevalence of occurrence or importance.

The procedures developed and used by Spitzer and his colleagues (1981) in developing the Quality-of-Life Index, or those recommended by Guyatt, Bombardier, and Tugwell (1986) for the development of disease-specific measures, ensure that validity of the content of the measures is firmly established.

## Reliability, Validity, and Responsiveness

Reliability, validity, and responsiveness are important properties of all instruments. Maintaining reliability is a quality control measure to ensure that the methods of the study are being employed as they should be. The validity of a measure is complex, but ultimately it is complete when the numbers from the summary score or the changes in scores have meaning for the persons using the information to make decisions. For the most part this stage has not yet been reached with quality-of-life measures. The thrust of health care is to maintain or improve the quality of life of individuals receiving services. The responsiveness of the instrument has to be sensitive to real changes in the health status of the individual that impinge on the quality of life. These three properties of instruments are discussed in detail in Chapter 6.

## Conclusions

Quality of life is becoming an important outcome variable in the evaluation of health care. Measures for it are now routinely employed in clinical trials of cancer treatment and in studies of heart disease, end-stage renal disease, palliative care, and rheumatoid arthritis.

A debate exists whether quality-of-life measures per se should be used for "ostensibly healthy" individuals such as might be found in family practices and other ambulatory care settings. Spitzer (1987) and Ware (1987) argue that functional status measures should be used in such settings. Others argue that such global measures as life satisfaction and subjective well-being are still in order here. The decision is that of the investigator, and the choice ultimately depends on the goals of the study.

Another issue arises in the study of quality of life. To this point most research is conducted to develop new measures or in the context of formal trials of interventions. A logical extension of the use of these measures would be to include them in assessments of quality of care. The Major Outcome Study (Stewart et al., 1988; Tarlov et al., 1989) is one step in this direction. Another is the work by Fowler and his colleagues (1988) to study the consequences of transuretheral prostatectomy.

In conclusion, researchers have been moving along two planes of activity; finding new uses in quality of life assessments for existing measures and developing new measures of quality of life. It is time to consolidate these activities and systematically advance the field. The emphasis should be on the scientific development and refinement of existing measures.

New ones should be created only when the list of available measures has been exhausted.

## References

Anderson, J. P., Bush, J. W., & Berry, C. C. (1988). Internal consistency analysis: A method for studying the accuracy of function assessment for health outcome and quality of life evaluation. *Journal of Clinical Epidemiology, 41*, 127-137.

Andrews, F. M., & Withey, S. B. (1976). *Social indicators of well-being: American perspectives of life quality.* New York: Plenum.

Bergner, M., Bobbit, R. A., Carter, W. B., & Gilson, B. S. (1981). The Sickness Impact Profile: Development and final revision of a health status measure. *Medical Care, 19*, 787-805.

Bradburn, N. M. (1969). *The structure of psychological well-being. Chicago: Aldine.*

Brook, R. H., Ware, J. E., Jr., Rogers W. H., Keeler, E. B., Davies, A. R., Donald, A. R., Goldberg, G. A., Lohr, K. N., Masthay, P. C., & Newhouse, J. P. (1983). Does free care improve adults' health? Results from a randomized controlled trial. *New England Journal of Medicine, 309*, 1426-1434.

Campbell, A. (1981). *The sense of well-being in America: Recent patterns and trends.* New York: McGraw-Hill.

Campbell, A., Converse, P. E., & Rodgers, W. (1976). *The quality of American life.* New York: Russell Sage.

Chambers, L. W. (1988). The McMaster Health Index Questionnaire: An update. In S. R. Walker & R. M. Rosser (Eds.), *Quality of life assessment and application* (pp. 131-132). Lancaster, England: MTP Press Ltd.

Chubon, R. A. (1985). Quality of life measurement of persons with back problems: Some preliminary findings. *Journal of Applied Rehabilitation Counselling, 16*, 31-34.

Chubon, R. A. (1986). Quality of life and persons with end-stage renal disease. *Dialysis and Transplantation, 15*, 450-452.

Chubon, R. A. (1987). A quality of life rating scale. *Evaluation and the Health Professions, 10*, 186-200.

Coates, A., Gebski, V., Bishop, J. F., Jeal, P. N., Woods, R. L., Snyder, R., Tattersall, M. H., Byrne, M., Harvey, V., & Gill, G. (1987). Improving the quality of life during chemotherapy for advanced breast cancer: A comparison of intermittent and continuous treatment strategies. *New England Journal of Medicine, 317*, 1490-1495.

Deyo, R. A., & Inui, T. S. (1984). Toward clinical applications of health status measures: Sensitivity of scales to clinically important changes. *Health Services Research, 19*, 275-289.

Dupuy, H. J. (1973). *Developmental rationale, substantive, derivative, and conceptual relevance of general well-being.* Washington, DC: National Center for Health Statistics.

Feinstein, A. R., Josephy, B. R., & Wells, C. K. (1986). Scientific and clinical problems in indexes of functional disability. *Annals of Internal Medicine, 105*, 413-420.

Ferrans, C. E., & Powers, M. J. (1985). Quality of Life Index: Development and psychometric properties. *Advances in Nursing Science, 8*, 15-24.

Finkelstein, D. M., Cassileth, B. R., Bonomi, P. D., Ruckdeschel, J. C., Ezdinli, E. Z., & Wolter, J. M. (1988). A pilot study of the Functional Living Index—Cancer (FLIC) Scale for the assessment of quality of life for metastatic lung cancer patients. *American Journal of Clinical Oncology, 2*, 630-633.

Fletcher, R. H., Fletcher, S. W., & Wagner, E. H. (1988). *Clinical epidemiology: The essentials* (2nd ed). Baltimore: Williams and Wilkins.

Fowler, F. J., Wennberg, J. E., Timothy, R. P., Barry, M. J., Mulley, A. G., Jr., & Hanley, D. (1988). Symptom status and quality of life following prostatectomy. *Journal of the American Medical Association, 259,* 3018-3022.

Guyatt, G. H., Bombardier, C., & Tugwell, P. X. (1986). Measuring disease-specific quality of life in clinical trials. *Journal of the Canadian Medical Association, 134,* 889-895.

Haynes, B. R. (1988). Selected principles of the measurement and setting of priorities of death, disability and suffering in clinical trials. *American Journal of Medical Sciences, 296,* 364-369.

Hollandsworth, J. G., Jr. (1988). Evaluating the impact of medical treatment on the quality of life: A 5-year update. *Social Science and Medicine, 26,* 425-434.

Hunt, S. M., McEwen, J., & McKenna, S. P. (1985). Measuring health status: A tool for clinicians and epidemiologists. *Journal of the Royal College of General Practice, 35,* 185-188.

Kaplan, R. M., Atkins, C. J., & Times, R. (1984). Validity of quality of well-being scale as an outcome measure in chronic obstructive pulmonary disease. *Journal of Chronic Diseases, 37,* 85-95.

Kaplan, R. W., & Bush, J. W. (1982). Health related quality of life measurement for evaluation research and policy analysis. *Health Psychology, 1,* 61-80.

Karnofsky, D. A., & Burchemal, J.H. (1949). The clinical evaluation of chemotherapeutic agents in cancer. In C. M. MacLeod (Ed.), *Evaluation of chemotherapeutic agents in cancer* (pp. 191-205). New York: Columbia University Press.

Lawton, M. P. (1975). The Philadelphia Geriatric Morale Scale: A revision. *Journal of Gerontology, 30,* 85-89.

Levine, M. N., Guyatt, G. H., Gent, M., et al. (1988). Quality of life in stage II breast cancer: An instrument for clinical trials. *Journal of Clinical Oncology, 6,* 1798-1810.

McNair, D. M., Lorr, M., & Drappleman, L. F. (1971). *EDITs manual for the profile of moods state.* San Diego: Educational and Industrial Testing Service.

Najman, J. M., & Levine, S. (1981). Evaluating the impact of medical care and technologies on the quality of life: A review and critique. *Social Science and Medicine, Part F: Medical and Social Ethics, 15F,* 107-115.

Neugarten, B., Havighurst, R., & Tobin, S. (1961). The measure of life satisfaction. *Journal of Gerontology, 16,* 134-143.

Padilla, G. V., & Grant, M. M. (1985). Quality of life as a cancer nursing outcome variable. *Advances in Nursing Science, 8,* 45-60.

Padilla, G. V., Presant, C., Grant, C., Metter, G., Lipsett, J., & Heide, F. (1983). Quality of life index for patients with cancer. *Research in Nursing and Health, 6,* 117-126.

Parkerson, G. R., Jr., Gehlback, S. H., Wagner, E. H., James, S. A., Clappin, N. E., & Muhlbaier, L. H. (1981). The Duke-UNC health profile: An adult health status instrument for primary care. *Medical Care, 19,* 806-828.

Parkerson, G. R., Jr., Michener, J. L., Wu, L. R., Finch, J. N., Muhlbaier, L. H., Magruder-Habib, K., Kertesz, J. W., Clapp-Channing, N., Morrow, D. S., Chen, A. L., et al. (1989). Associations among family support, family stress, and personal functional health status. *Journal of Clinical Epidemiology, 42,* 217-229.

Raghavan, D., Grundy, R., & Lancaster, L. (1988). Assessment of quality of life in long-term survivors treated by first-line intravenous cisplating for invasive bladder cancer. *Progress in Clinical and Biological Research, 260,* 625-631.

Rosenberg, M. (1962). *Society and the adolescent self-image.* Princeton, NJ: Princeton University Press.

Schipper, H., Clinch, J., McMurray, A., & Levitt, M. (1984). Measuring the quality of life of cancer patients: The Functional Living Index—Cancer: Development and validation. *Journal of Clinical Oncology, 2*, 472-483.

Spitzer, W. O. (1987). State of science 1986: Quality of life and functional status as target variables for research. *Journal of Chronic Diseases, 40*, 465-471.

Spitzer, W. O., Dobson, A. J., Hall, J., Chesterman, E., Levi, J., Shepherd, R., Battista, R. N., & Catchlove, B. R. (1981). Measuring the quality of life of cancer patients: A concise QL-index for use by physicians. *Journal of Chronic Diseases, 34*, 585-597.

Stewart, A. L., Hays, R. D., & Ware, J. E., Jr. (1988). The MOS short form general health survey: Reliability and validity in a patient population. *Medical Care, 26*, 724-735.

Tarlov, A. R., Ware, J. E., Jr., Greenfield, S., Nelson, E. C., Perrin, E., & Zubkoff, M. (1989). The medical outcomes study: An application of methods for monitoring the results of medical care. *Journal of the American Medical Association, 262*, 925-930.

Torrance, G. W. (1982). Multiattribute utility theory as a method for measuring social preferences for health care states in long-term care. In R. L. Kane & R. A. Kane (Eds.), *Values and long-term care* (pp. 127-156). Toronto: Lexington.

Torrance, G. W. (1986). Measurement of health state utilities for economic appraisal: A review. *Journal of Health Economics, 3*, 1-30.

Torrance, G. W. (1987). Utility approach to measuring health-related quality of life. *Journal of Chronic Diseases, 40*, 593-600.

Torrance, G. W., Boyle, M. H., & Horwood, S. P. (1982). Application of multiattribute utility theory to measure social preferences for health states. *Operations Research, 30*, 1043-1069.

Torrance, G. W., Thomas, W. H., & Sackett, D. L. (1972). A utility maximization model for the evaluation of health care programs. *Health Services Research, 7*, 118-133.

von Neumann, J., & Morgenstern, O. (1953). *Theory of games and economic behavior* (3rd ed.). New York: John Wiley.

Wallston, K. A., Kaplan, G. D., & Maides, S. A. (1976). Development and validation of Health Locus of Control (HLC) scale. *Journal of Consulting Clinical Psychology, 44*, 580-585.

Ware, J. E., Jr. (1987). Standards for validating health measures: Definition and content. *Journal of Chronic Diseases, 40*, 473-480.

Ware, J. E., Jr., Manning, W. G., Jr., Duan, N., et al. (1984). Health status and the use of ambulatory mental health services. *American Psychologist, 39*, 1090-1100.

Weinstein, M. C., Fineberg, H. V., Elstein, A. S., Frazier, H. S., Newhauser, D., Neutra, R. R., & NcNeil, B. J. (1980). *Clinical decision analysis* (pp. 184-227). Philadelphia, PA: W. B. Saunders.

Williams, J. I., & Wood-Dauphinee, S. (1989). Assessing quality of life: Measures and utility. In F. Mosteller & J. Falotico-Taylor (Eds.), *Quality of life and technology assessment* (pp. 65-115). Washington, DC: National Academy of Science.

# 12  Family Assessment Measures

CINDY I. CARLSON

## Introduction

Increasingly, primary care physicians are becoming aware of the role that family plays in illness and health. In addition to genetic factors, patterns of social relationships among family members can either increase an individual's risk and vulnerability to disease or conversely provide a buffer that strengthens the resilience of vulnerable persons. Given the onset of disease, the family system's competence as health care providers will affect recovery. In addition many bodily symptoms or complaints reflect psychosomatic disorders that can be indicative of family conflict or stress. Thus an orientation by the primary care physician to all these aspects can provide information critical to the selection of an intervention.

This chapter introduces primary care physicians to the range and limitations of various methods and measures in family assessment. The theoretical foundation and goals are presented first, followed by a discussion of two main types of assessment—observational and self-report methods. The last part discusses issues to consider in the selection of an instrument. It is beyond the scope of this chapter to describe and evaluate specific measures: the interested reader is referred to Grotevant and Carlson (1989); Touliatos, Perlmutter, and Straus (1989); and Filsinger (1983).

## Conceptual Foundations

Measures of family functioning derive from diverse theoretical bases and disciplines of inquiry. Whatever the lens through which it is being viewed, however, an assessment of the family context typically is largely driven by adoption of a *systems framework* (Steinglass, 1987). A *system* is defined as "a series of elements arranged in some consistent and enduring relationship with each other." In addition to this definition, which emphasizes the internal organizational properties of systems, *biological systems* are defined as "living or *open* systems" because they cannot grow and differentiate without the input of energy from the environment. The systems perspective provides an organismic approach to disease in which pathology is viewed not as a linear cause-and-effect reaction but rather in terms of malfunctioning interactions between factors or components within a system or between the system and its environment. Disease signals a breakdown of customary regulatory processes, such that the optimal organization of the organism's internal environment is undermined and must be restored. Clinical implications of a systems perspective are (a) that organisms and their symptoms, when not viewed within their social context, may be unrecognizable; and (b) that a correction of pathology in one part of the system may have unintended consequences for related elements within or surrounding the system.

The application of a systems perspective to the family defines it as an organized unit comprised of elements (individuals) and subunits (e.g., parents, children) existing in some enduring, consistent relationship with one another. The organization of these elements and subunits are patterned—not random—and hierarchical. Thus assessment of the family system implies attention to the patterns and organization of the elements that characterize the whole of its milieu. The enduring, consistent relationships among family members are evident in their repeated transactional patterns with one another and, since the family is a living system, with the world at large (Minuchin, 1974). This coherence may be evident also in the subjective evaluations that family members hold of one another, of their relationships with each other, of the family as a whole, and of their orientation toward the environment (see, for example, Reiss, 1981).

Defining the family as a system and its members as elements of this system implies that these members, regardless of motivation, will be either constrained or enabled in their individual behavior and development by the nature of the relationships they have with each other. This influence has directed the attention of family researchers and clinicians to the role that individual symptomatology may play within a family. From this perspective, symptoms may reflect one of the following: (a) an adaptation to a dysfunctional system, (b) an attempt to maintain homeostasis of the family system of a subsystem, (c) a protective mechanism for the symptom-bearer, or (d) a rigid complementarity within the family. Viewed in this manner, the symptom of obesity, for example, might (a) reflect a depressive response to perceived rejection by one's spouse, (b) serve to maintain emotional distance between the marital couple, (c) protect the obese individual from anxiety-producing behaviors (e.g., gaining employment), or (d) serve as the essential counterbalance to an overtly negative and critical but emotionally insecure spouse. Treatment of the obesity without consideration of the family relationships in which the patient is embedded is likely to fail.

Viewed differently, defining the family as an open system implies that the injury or disease of one member will affect the roles and relationships of all. As noted by Minuchin (1974), a family is subject both to inner pressure coming from developmental changes in its own members and to outer pressures coming from demands to accommodate the social institutions that have an impact on it. Acute or chronic illness of a family member increases both types of demands: Internally it requires an adaptation by other members of their roles and expectations; externally, in this age of specialized medicine, it typically demands interaction with multiple health care settings and personnel. Thus a key focus of family assessment in health-related research and practice is how members deal with stress and coping.

The widespread adoption of a systems perspective for conceptualizing families has resulted in the identification of common organizational properties. Two of these have been mentioned already: the family's coping ability or adaptability, and the homeostatic role of symptoms within it. Additional ones include the quality of family structure, roles, hierarchy, complementarity, boundaries, communications, affect, and goodness-of-fit.

The *structure*, or organization, of the family is "the invisible set of functional demands that organizes the ways in which family members interact" (Minuchin, 1974, p. 51). Families can be viewed as organizations with multiple tasks to accomplish, including for example, the provision of shelter, economic security, safety, child care, emotional support, home maintenance, leisure and recreation, and sexual satisfaction. In order to accomplish these many roles, family systems must be organized into subunits, with a clear hierarchy of authority and complementarity of functions. Thus for the family to maintain itself it must be adequately organized to carry out everyday functions without undue stress and conflict. On the other hand it must be flexible enough to adapt when circumstances change.

The rules governing the organization of the family are evident when viewing the repeated transactions that occur among its members. Those rules that define who can participate in what activities are also termed the *boundaries* between individuals and subunits of the family. Boundaries serve to protect the differentiation of the family system; for example, individual members or subsystems are not placed in a position in which they must enact roles that are inappropriate to their age or developmental level. Incest, for example, signifies weak boundaries between the subsystems of parent and child; parental overprotection of a sickly child in a way that compromises the child's development of autonomy would also be viewed as signaling inadequate boundaries. Families with clear boundaries—that is, repeated patterns of transaction that convey clear rules about the appropriate behavior of each member based on family values and individual developmental levels—are viewed as being the most functional.

Although the concept of a boundary brings to mind the idea of a barrier, the boundaries within a family are viewed as permeable, in that while they protect members from noxious elements that would compromise their health, they are permeable to the passage of essential, growth-producing "nutrients." The nutrients of families are *communication* of information and sharing of *affect*. Thus another focus of family assessment is frequently the quality of the communication between the members, and the degree to which evidence exists of an appropriate level of affective involvement.

Finally it is important to note that although the family as a system has universal features, an assessment of its functioning must also consider the developmental needs of individual members, the stressors currently experienced by the family, and the demands and values of the sociocultural milieu. The presence of individual symptomatology, when psychogenic in origin, is considered suggestive of possible difficulty on the part of family members in reorganizing their roles to meet one another's changing needs or the demands of the external world.

In summary, assessment of family functioning is rooted firmly in the conceptual framework of general systems theory, which argues the interrelatedness of elements, their organization into patterns, and the principle of nonsummativity (that is, the whole is greater than the sum of its parts). Consistent with this theory, family assessment methods focus measurement and analysis on the patterns of relationship organization that characterize the whole family as a unit. Measurement of a whole that reflects the unique patterning of subunits has posed considerable methodological challenge to family researchers. These methodological issues will be addressed near the end of the chapter; first, the various forms of family assessment will be discussed.

## Types of Family Assessment

### OBSERVATIONAL METHODS

Observational methods permit the direct assessment of family interaction patterns. Appreciation for the value of this approach has increased in recent decades due to a variety of factors: (a) the emphasis of many current theories of family therapy on here-and-now interactions rather than history, (b) the questionable validity of self-report measures, and (c) technological and psychometric advances that have improved the feasibility of collecting and analyzing observational data. Observational methods are of three main types: interview procedures, clinical rating scales, and coding schemes. These can be viewed as ranging on a continuum from informal to formal, nonstandardized to standardized, clinical to scientific, unreliable to reliable, or subjective to objective.

Observation methods also can vary in the degree of observer participation: that is, the extent to which the observer is clearly visible to the individuals being observed. An observer may maintain a passive, noninteractive role, such as when trained coders note interactions within the home setting; or may be involved in interaction with the family, such as during a clinical interview (Margolin, 1987). (Participant observation sometimes also refers to situations in which family members are directed to monitor the behaviors of each other; however, for the purposes of this chapter these will be considered as self-report methods.)

Because it is recognized that the observer's objectivity is influenced by participation in the interaction with the family members and by the history of his or her association with them (Margolin, 1987), several techniques have been developed to aid in the validity and reliability of these data. The most frequently used include interview procedures and clinical rating scales.

*Interview Procedures.* Participant observation of family interactions during a clinical interview is the espoused method of assessment by models that focus diagnosis on family transactions occurring in the here and now. An informal participant observation might direct attention, for example, to the quality of boundaries, hierarchy, emotional closeness, and clarity of communication among members. In order to ensure that transactions of theoretical or clinical interest are likely to occur, some family treatment models have developed interview procedures to aid in informal clinical evaluation, and several have developed interview procedures to be used in conjunction with clinical rating scales (e.g., Skinner's Family Process Model [1983]; Olson's Circumplex Model of Family Functioning [1986]).

The interview procedure is also useful for eliciting and evaluating individuals' subjective beliefs about their family, such as attitudes and attributions, relationships, or a particular family member or problem. Procedures focusing on cognitions are best developed by cognitive-behavioral family therapists (Epstein, Baldwin, & Bishop, 1983).

Informal observation of family functioning during an interview has both distinct advantages and disadvantages for primary care research. The primary advantage is low cost, as this technique can be incorporated relatively easily into a practice. The primary disadvantage, of course, is the lack of objectivity, validity, and reliability of data that derive from the observer's clinical judgment, even if he or she is well trained. Thus informal participant observation alone is unlikely to be useful as a research methodology in primary care unless a second observer is included, so that interrater reliability can be determined, and the aid of a measurement technique is used, such as a checklist or rating scale.

*Clinical Rating Scales.* Clinical rating scales are a family assessment technique designed to permit a summary judgment on the part of the rater/observer with regard to placement of an individual, dyad, or entire family on some psychological dimension. Such scales are useful either following an interview as a means of recording impressions in a more standardized fashion, or in a nonparticipant observation of the family in interaction (for example, from behind a one-way mirror or from video recordings). The advantages include cost efficiency, generation of data that can be evaluated for reliability and validity, and communication with other professionals.

The usefulness of clinical rating scales, however, is largely constrained by two factors: rater competence, and the psychometric quality of the scale. These scales require raters to use their complex information-processing capabilities to make summary judgments on particular dimensions of the family; however, the varying capacity of the raters to integrate diverse information has contributed to the lack of reliability. For reliable ratings the following assumptions must hold (Cairns & Green, 1979):

1. Raters share with the author of the scale and with other raters a theoretical concept of the quality or attribute to be rated.
2. Raters share a concept of which behaviors reflect that quality or attribute.
3. Raters are able to detect information relevant to the attribute in the stream of behavior.
4. Raters share the same underlying psychometric "scale" on which the attribute will be judged.
5. Raters have sufficient knowledge about the comparison or reference group to place the observed behavior on a distribution.

These abilities are enhanced, of course, with rater training, as well as by careful construction of the rating scale. Rating scales that have clearly defined and behaviorally defined anchor points, equal psychological distance between anchor points, and an adequate number of anchor points increase the likelihood that ratings will be reliable. For additional discussion of rater errors and an evaluation of existing clinical rating scales of family functioning, see Carlson and Grotevant (1987) and Grotevant and Carlson (1989).

*Coding Schemes.* The most objective and scientific observation method of family assessment involves the use of a family interaction *coding scheme.* Coding schemes refer to the precise recording of the precise actions of individuals in a group, the analysis of which is essential for understanding the processes of interaction (Grotevant & Carlson, 1987, 1989). This technique has many research advantages. Coding schemes require fewer inferences, are less susceptible to confounding influences, have greater face validity and generalizability, preserve the actions of family members for multiple analyses, are flexible in providing quantitative indices, can be used by nonprofessionals, and have enhanced reliability. In short they provide the most "objective" view of the family, and research aimed at determining the contingent patterns of interaction within families typically requires them as the primary method of data collection.

On the negative side, however, many of the characteristics of the family interaction coding schemes that enhance their objectivity also create limitations. They are typically more costly to apply than other methods even with the availability of advanced technology. Their higher cost frequently limits their application to a single session, which may be unrepresentative of the family's behavior. Moreover, to enhance reliability, codings of family interaction usually require consistency of the task, setting, number, and role of family members. Another limitation is their microanalytic perspective. The precise recording of actions and reactions among family members requires a limited number and scope of behavioral codes; every decision to limit the scope of behavior to be coded is likely to enhance reliability and to afford greater power in data analysis but at the cost of comprehensiveness. In short, coding schemes are well suited to investigations of well-focused, theoretically based research based on the contingent behaviors of individuals within family relationships but may not be ideal for capturing qualities of the whole system.

One solution to these limitations is to change the level of analysis at which behavior is coded and analyzed; that is, change the focus of the coding behavior and unit from an individual to a dyad or the whole family. This approach appears to have considerable merit for researchers

in validating theoretical models of family functioning based on rela-
tional patterns of interaction (Grotevant & Carlson, 1989).

## ISSUES IN OBSERVATION

A number of issues should be considered in the use of observation as
a method of family assessment, primarily having to do with the reliability and validity of the data. Reliability is most strongly affected by coder
training, coder drift, and the clarity of the constructs. A number of
methods of determining interrater reliability of observation data can be
used; the use of Cohen's kappa statistic is most frequently recommended, as it corrects for chance agreement between raters (Grotevant
& Carlson, 1989; Touliatos et al., 1989). In selecting a family interaction
coding scheme, the recommended acceptable Cohen's kappa reliability
range is .60 to .75 (Hartmann, 1982).

The reliability of a coding scheme, of course, constrains validity. For
observation methods, three types of validity are relevant: content validity, criterion-related validity, and construct validity. A review of existing
family interaction coding schemes has found that although promising
validation efforts have been made, the high cost of data collection and
analysis, as well as the tendency of researchers to create new codes
for their own purposes, makes for limited within-method comparisons
(Grotevant & Carlson, 1989). Identical behaviors are represented sometimes with different constructs, and vice versa. A review of family
clinical rating scales also finds evidence of validity to be emerging but
incomplete, primarily accounted for by the newness of these measures
(Carlson & Grotevant, 1987).

In addition to concerns about reliability and validity, several other
potential sources of invalidity in the use of observation methods must
be considered. These include the setting, task, reactivity, and recording
of the observation, all of which may alter the pattern of family interaction that is desired by the researcher. Laboratory settings, for example,
may constrain negative interactions. Similarly, if the focus of the research is family conflict, it will be essential to develop a procedure and
task that elicit conflict. Both the presence of the observer and the intru-
siveness of the recording procedure are also likely to affect interactions.
Thus the researcher has numerous decisions to consider in the selection
of an existing coding scheme or the creation of a new one. (For additional
discussion see Grotevant & Carlson, 1989).

## SELF-REPORT METHODS

In contrast with observation methods of family assessment, which are considered to provide an "outsider" perspective of the functioning (Olson, 1986), self-report methods provide an "insider" view. For the purposes of this chapter, *self-report measures* are defined as "standardized questionnaires that provide information about individual family members' subjective reality or experiences, including perceptions of self and other family members, attitudes regarding family (roles, values, etc.), and satisfaction with relationships." (As noted earlier, directives to some family members to record the behavior of others may also be considered self-report methods. Since these methods are seldom focused on the family as a unit, they are not considered further here. The interested reader is referred to Margolin (1987) for a discussion of this approach.)

Self-report measures were the predominant methodology in studies of the family through the 1970s; however, their reliability and validity as objective measures of behavior were seriously challenged (Grotevant & Carlson, 1989). Currently interest has renewed in this approach. First, methods for evaluating respondents' biases have been developed, which increase validity. Perhaps more significant, however, has been the increased recognition of the diagnostic and research significance of the individual's subjective reality as a predictor of his or her behavior with others. Thus, with the growing popularity of family systems theory, numerous self-report measures have been developed. For purposes of the primary care physician/researcher, these may be categorized broadly as measures of family functioning and measures of family stress and coping.

*Family Functioning Measures.* Self-report measures of family functioning refer to questionnaires designed to assess the quality of relationships within the family or characteristics of the family milieu that are reflective of healthy functioning. In a recent review of 17 measures of whole family functioning (Grotevant & Carlson, 1989), it was determined that most of these measures were compatible with family systems theory; however, the scope of assessment varied widely. Four key dimensions of family functioning were identified: structure, process, affect, and orientation. Only 3 of the 17 measures were found actually to assess all four dimensions: Emery, Weintraub, and Neale (1980); Roelofse and Middleton (1985); and Skinner & Steinhauer (1986). Comprehensiveness, of course, may not be the researcher's goal; rather the theoretical compatibility of a measure is underscored. With regard to this, these reviewers noted the importance of looking beyond the names of scales of self-report measures to actual item content, as several inconsistencies were noted in the issues assessed by scales that have the same name. For example, in one measure "expressiveness in the family" referred to the exchange of ideas, whereas in another it referred to the sharing of feeling. In conclusion these reviewers noted that the lack of clarity and the theoretical diversity among the existing self-report measures points to a lack of theoretical consensus. The prospective researcher is cautioned to conduct a careful examination of a measure prior to use in research.

*Family Stress and Coping.* A second focus of self-report measures addresses the family's capacity to cope with stress. These measures appear to be of particular salience to primary care researchers who may be interested in the resilience or vulnerability of individuals or family units in the face of inordinate stressors. A recent review of this area identified nine measures (Grotevant & Carlson, 1989). Most of these were derived theoretically from either sociological family theory or family systems theory, which focuses on the whole family as a unit, and were consistent with the family stress literature, which acknowledges the relationship between the variables of adaptive functioning, coping strategies, and sources of social support in the family. As with the findings of the review of measures of family functioning, the measures in this area are notable for construct inconsistency, and only one could be considered comprehensive: Sawa, Falk, and Pablo (1986). At present it would appear that the primary care researcher would need to use multiple measures to gain an assessment perspective that matched the breadth of family stress theory. As noted by the reviewers, the need to use multiple measures increases the complexity of the researcher's interpretive task and requires careful examination of the interrelations among measures. In addition many of the measures reviewed lacked studies of criterion-related or construct validity. For the most part their value remains uncertain. This area is one that will benefit greatly by additional research.

ISSUES IN SELF-REPORT

Attention to the reliability and validity of any measurement device is always essential for the researcher. Since the assessment of validity for self-report measures is similar to that for observation methods, the focus here will be on threats to reliability that are unique to questionnaires. One of the reasons why self-report measures fell out of favor in the 1970s was the discovery that a variety of response set biases have the potential for introducing systematic error into scores. These threats to reliability include respondents answering in a socially desirable manner, including faking good, defensiveness, and lying, as well as faking bad or malingering; lack of semantic clarity in the question; situational effects, which may bias responses; or lack of self-awareness on the part of the respondent. A number of strategies have been developed to reduce or test for the effect of response sets; these should be incorporated into the development of self-report questionnaires (see Nunnally, 1978).

Another issue is the discrepancy between the unit of *perception*—that is, the subjective evaluation of an individual family member—and the unit of *inquiry*, which is the whole family unit. The extent to which an individual respondent can provide useful information about variables in the system is an important consideration in deciding whether to use this method in family research. Self-report measures are the method of choice only when the research question concerns the attitudes and comparisons of different family members' points of view; they cannot be used as a true indicator of the perception of the whole family.

The derivation of a family unit score is controversial among researchers. Some researchers create it by pooling and averaging scores across the individual members. This strategy, however, rests on the assumption that all members' perceptions are equally valid and also can distort important deviations on the part of a single member from others in the family. Another approach to the problem of multiple perceptions is to derive measures of concordance among family members—called *discrepancy scores* or *ratio scores*. The primary disadvantage of these scores is their failure to locate the individual, couple, or family on a particular dimension. Researchers, therefore, frequently are advised to use both average and discrepancy scores to coordinate individual data into family unit scores (Larsen & Olson, 1990).

In summary, self-report measures of family functioning and family stress and coping are useful methods for the assessment of individual members' subjective evaluations of each other. Although these measures purport to look at the whole family unit and utilize constructs that are in fact consistent with systems theory, in reality (unless completed by the whole family together) they can be considered only to be measures of individuals. The creation of family scores based on some combination of individual members' data is the obvious solution that has been provided for this problem; however, the differential weights that may be appropriate for a given member's perspective, and the meaning of unique combinations of individual scores, remain questions to be answered by future empirical research.

## Summary and Conclusion:
## Issues in Family Assessment

Interest in family measurement has increased considerably in recent decades as evidenced both by the development of numerous measures and a plethora of theories from diverse disciplines. As noted by Larzelere and Klein (1986), however, "*What* we know about families is largely determined by *how* we know what we know" (p. 125). This chapter has focused on how researchers can come to know about families, and the limitations that each particular lens affords. Several themes have emerged that deserve highlighting.

Psychometric quality is a concern that must remain central to the primary care physician or researcher in the selection of any assessment measure. Significant progress has been made in the validation of observation and self-report methods; however, some areas, such as family stress and coping, appear to lag in maturity and deserve particular attention. Moreover few measures have adequate normative data for comparison in research, and fewer still have adequate norms for clinical use.

Another concern in this field is the lack of a theoretical consensus regarding family process or functioning. Cowan (1987) has suggested that we may be putting the cart before the horse if we continue to focus on the development of reliable measures before facilitating the development of theories out of which they must emerge. What are the implications of this for primary care researchers? One is that research directed toward theory development and validation is important. A second is that when selecting a measure, one must pay careful attention to the theory base from which it is developed and to its actual item content (whether self-report items or observation codes). Correspondence of constructs across measures cannot be assumed. Finally, theoretical perspective will influence the researcher's data analysis decisions; for example, the construction of family scores from individual self-report, or cluster versus sequential analysis of interaction data.

The complexity of theoretical and methodological issues here points also to a central concern: the determination of the level and unit of analysis. The systems theory principle of nonsummativity emphasizes measurement of the whole family unit; however, researchers continue to find this a challenge for both observation codes and self-report measures. Moreover, evidence exists that assessment at each subsystem level of the family (e.g., individual, parent-child, spousal, sibling) adds unique information to our understanding of family phenomena that is not captured by one superordinate measurement (Carlson, Cooper, & Spradling, in press; Cowan, 1987). This possibility suggests that researchers who truly want to capture the family must engage in measurement at multiple levels or be clear in the focus of their inquiry on a specific subunit of the family system.

A final issue is the goal of research in this field. Primary care research combines scientific inquiry and clinical practice, and these two orientations may have different implications for selection of an instrument (Carlson, 1989). Two aspects of family assessment are highlighted in research: the degree to which identified abstract concepts have some rational and empirical correspondence with reality (validity), and the creation of good rules that permit empirical testing (reliability). In the clinical context, assessment refers to the careful analysis of clients such that an appropriate intervention may be selected; thus methods must be validated on their adequacy in meeting the sequential decision-making step of diagnosis, treatment, and evaluation. Of course any single device may have excellent validity for one phase of clinical treatment but not for others. For example, a measure designed for screening may be inadequate in detecting subtle changes in family interaction patterns. A review of existing family assessment measures suggests that few have been developed with the multiple functions of assessment in the clinical context in mind.

The distinctiveness of the needs of researchers and clinicians raises several recommendations for future work (Carlson, 1989). First, the purpose of a family assessment measure must be stated clearly so that the most salient features of its reliability and validity can be evaluated. Second, if measurement is related to treatment, then the nature of change should be specified theoretically and psychometrically so that reliability can be appropriately addressed. Third, continuous inquiry into the nature of multiple family respondents appears warranted. Finally, it would appear that the discrepancies often found in multilevel, multimethod assessments of the family have been poorly specified theoretically.

# References

Cairns, R. B., & Green, J. A. (1979). Appendix A: How to assess personality and social patterns. In R. B. Cairns (Ed.), *The analysis of social interactions: Methods, issues and illustrations* (pp. 209-255). Hillsdale, NJ: Lawrence Erlbaum.

Carlson, C. I. (1989). Criteria for family assessment. In H. D. Grotevant (Ed.), Current issues in marital and family assessment [Special issue]. *Journal of Family Psychology, 3*(2), 158-176.

Carlson, C. I., Cooper, C. R., & Spradling, V. Y. (in press). Developmental implications of shared vs. distinct perceptions of the family in early adolescence. In R. L. Paikoff (Ed.), *Shared views in the family during adolescence.* San Francisco: Jossey-Bass.

Carlson, C. I., & Grotevant, H. D. (1987). A comparative review of family rating scales: Guidelines for clinicians and researchers. *Journal of Family Psychology, 1*(1), 23-47.

Cowan, P. A. (1987). The need for theoretical and methodological integrations in family research. *Journal of Family Psychology, 1*(1), 48-50.

Emery, R. E., Weintraub, S., & Neale, J. M. (1980, August). *The family evaluation form: Construction and normative data.* Paper presented at the annual meeting of the American Psychological Association, Montreal.

Epstein, N. B., Baldwin, L. M., & Bishop, D. (1983). The McMaster family assessment device. *The Journal of Marital and Family Therapy, 9*(2), 171-180.

Filsinger, E. E. (1983). *Marriage and family assessment.* Beverly Hills, CA: Sage.

Grotevant, H. D., & Carlson, C. I. (1989). *Family assessment: A guide to methods and measures.* New York: Guilford.

Hartmann, D. P (Ed.). (1982). *Using observers to study behavior: New directions for methodology of social and behavior science.* San Francisco: Jossey-Bass.

Larsen, A., & Olson, D. (1990). Capturing the complexity of family systems: Integrating family theory, family scores, and family analysis. In T. W. Draper & A. C. Marcos (Eds.), *Family variables: Conceptualization, measurement, and use* (pp. 19-47). Beverly Hills, CA: Sage.

Larzelere, R. E., & Klein, D. M. (1986). Methodology. In M. B. Sussman & S. K. Steinmatz (Eds.), *Handbook of marriage and family* (pp.125-155). New York: Plenum.

Margolin, G. (1987). Participant observation procedures in marital and family assessment. In T. Jacob (Ed.), *Family interaction and psychopathology* (pp. 391-426). New York: Plenum.

Minuchin, S. (1974). *Families and family therapy.* Cambridge, MA: Harvard University Press.

Nunnally, J. C. (1978). *Psychometric theory* (2nd ed.). New York: McGraw-Hill.

Olson, D. H. (1986). Circumplex model VII: Validation studies and FACES III. *Family Process, 25,* 337-351.

Reiss, D. (1981). *The family's construction of reality.* Cambridge, MA: Harvard University Press.

Roelofse, R., & Middleton, M. R. (1985). The family functioning in adolescence questionnaire: A measure of psychosocial family health during adolescence. *Journal of Adolescence, 8,* 33-45.

Sawa, R. J., Falk, W. A., & Pablo, R. Y. (1986). *Assessing the family in primary care.* Unpublished manuscript.

Skinner, H., Steinhauer, P. D., & Santa-Barbara, J. (1983). The family assessment measure. *Canadian Journal of Community Mental Health, 2*(2), 91-105.

Steinglass, P. (1987). A systems view of family interaction and psychopathology. In T. Jacob (Ed.), *Family interaction and psychopathology* (pp.25-66). New York: Plenum.

Touliatos, J., Perlmutter, B. F., & Straus, M. A. (Eds.). (1989). *Handbook of family measurement techniques.* Beverly Hills, CA: Sage.

# 13 COOP Measures of Functional Status

DAVID W. BEAUFAIT
EUGENE C. NELSON
JEANNE M. LANDGRAF
RONALD D. HAYS
JOHN W. KIRK
JOHN H. WASSON
ADAM KELLER

A rich collection of measures exists on how patients feel, function, and perceive their own health. To comprehensively assess all of these aspects, however, requires extensive time on the part of patients, and elaborate scoring procedures. Although such measures are extremely valuable for large-scale research that needs highly sensitive assessments, they are not practical for the individual physician in dealing with patients in everyday office practice. Further, long-form surveys are not practical in studies that cannot afford extensive data collection.

Thus we provide in this chapter a very brief method for measuring function and health, which may be useful for routine use in clinical practice and practice-based research: the COOP Chart System. This system has been tested in scores of different practices, in both North America and elsewhere, to evaluate its validity, reliability, and acceptability (Nelson et al., 1987; Nelson et al., 1990a; Nelson, Wasson, & Kirk, 1987). WONCA is conducting a pilot test on these charts in approximately 20 countries, and the charts are being used in a major clinical trial in case-finding at the Harvard Community Health Plan and to measure quality of care by the Hospital Corporation of America. This chapter describes the COOP Chart System and the results of an evaluation of its reliability, validity, acceptability, and utility.

## The COOP Chart System

Many validated measures of health status are available (McDowell & Newell, 1987), but the vast majority are not suitable for office practice because they require too much time to administer and score. The COOP Chart System was developed by the Dartmouth COOP Project, a network of community practices that cooperate on research activities, specifically for use in office practices. It is based on the following six design principles:

1. It should produce reliable and valid data on a core set of dimensions of function and well-being.
2. It should be acceptable to patients, physicians, and office staff.
3. It should be applicable to a wide range of problems and diagnoses.
4. It should possess a high degree of face validity.
5. It should yield easily interpretable scores.
6. It should provide the practitioner with clinically useful information regarding a patient's functioning and well-being.

The COOP system consists of nine charts: the five original ones, which measure physical, social, and role functioning, emotional status, and overall health; two that were developed based on clinician interest in measuring pain and change in health; and two based on researcher interest on social support and quality of life. Three of the charts focus on specific dimensions of function, two on symptoms or feelings, three on perceptions, and one is a health covariate (see Figures 13.1 and 13.2).

The COOP charts are similar in their simplicity to Snellen charts used to measure visual acuity. Each consists of a simple title, a straightforward stem question regarding the patient's status on the relevant dimension over the past 4 weeks, and five response choices. Each response choice is illustrated by a drawing that depicts a level of functioning or well-being along a 5-point ordinal scale. In accordance with clinical convention, high scores represent unfavorable levels of health. Except for the overall health change chart, change can be coded as better (+), the same (0) or worse (–), in addition to the numerical score. Figures 13.1 and 13.2 show the nine charts.

## Source of Chart Contents

Many excellent methods of measuring function preceded the development of the COOP charts and were used as models for some of the charts' features, including prior COOP research (Nelson et al., 1983), the Rand Mental Health Inventory (Ware, Johnston, Davies-Avery, & Brook, 1979), the Katz ADL Index (Katz, Ford, Moskowitz, Jackson, & Jaffe, 1963), and the Goldman Specific Activity Scale (Goldman, Hashimoto, Cook, & Loscalzo, 1981). These all were designed for use in medical practice and are simple to administer, score, and interpret. Although the ADL index is most appropriate for long-term care patients with extensive limitations in physical functioning, it is not appropriate for ambulatory patients who have higher levels of physical ability. The New York Heart Association's measure, while popular and easy to use, focuses on limitations due to heart problems and has been shown to be unreliable (Goldman et al., 1981).

In other respects the charts resemble some of the best multidimensional measures of function, such as the Sickness Impact Profile (Bergner et al., 1976), the Duke-UNC Health Profile (Parkerson et al., 1981), the McMaster Health Index (Sackett, Chambers, MacPherson, Goldsmith, & Macauley, 1977), the Nottingham Health Profile (Hunt, McEwen, & McKennan, 1985), and the health status measures developed at RAND (Ware, 1987). All of these measures are multidimensional (that is, they assess physical, mental, and social function) and have been subjected to careful methodological studies to determine their reliability and validity.

In addition to these earlier instruments, the content of each chart came from expert advice from clinicians and health measurement professionals and went through several iterations before assuming its current form. This development process should therefore ensure a high degree of content validity.

## Methods of Administration

The COOP charts have been designed to fit into the standard data collection routine of busy ambulatory practices. They can be administered via two modes: provider-administered (physician, nurse, medical assistant), or patient self-administered.

For the first method the patient is shown the charts one at a time and is asked to read the question carefully and to indicate the answer that best depicts his or her status. Scores are recorded in the patient's medical record, on a flow sheet, or in the progress note for that visit, using self-adhesive labels. Careful administration technique is necessary to avoid influencing responses.

The second method utilizes the time spent by the patient in the waiting area of the practitioner's office, with the patient reading and completing a patient packet containing the charts and an answer sheet. Each chart

(Text continues on p. 158)

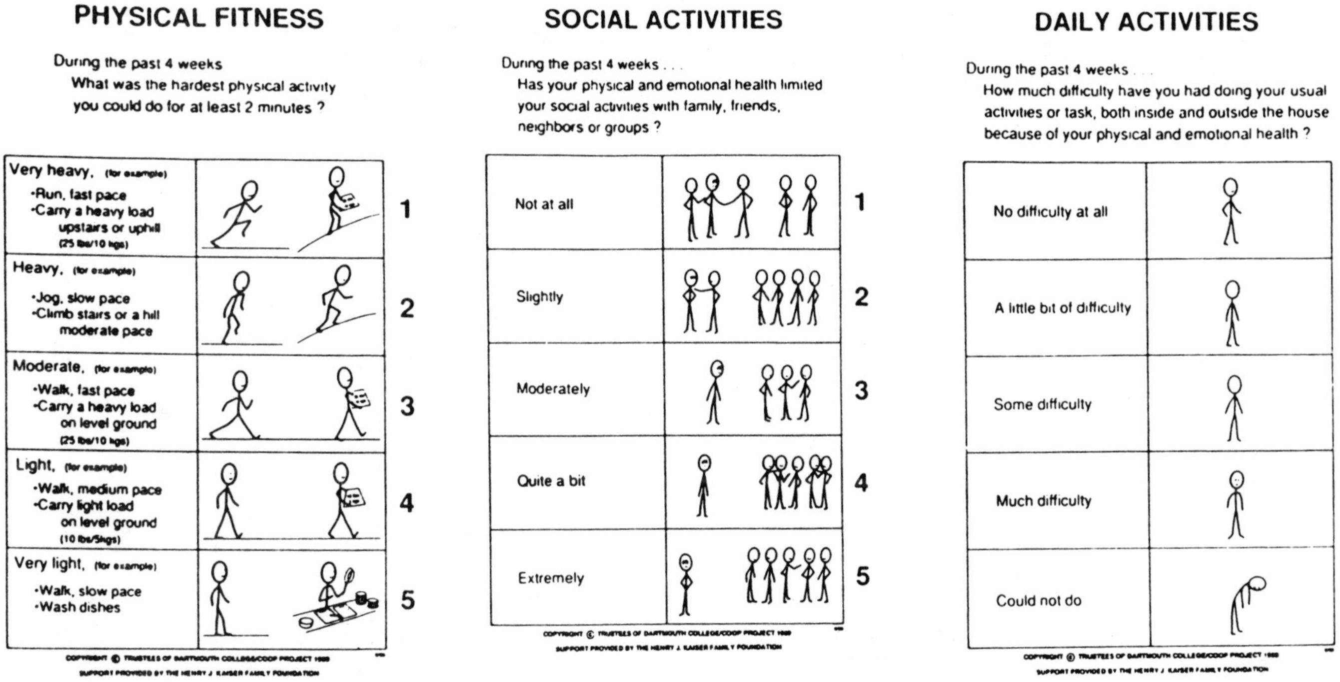

**Figure 13.1.** Five of the Nine COOP Charts: Physical Fitness, Social Activities, Daily Activities, Feelings, and Overall Health

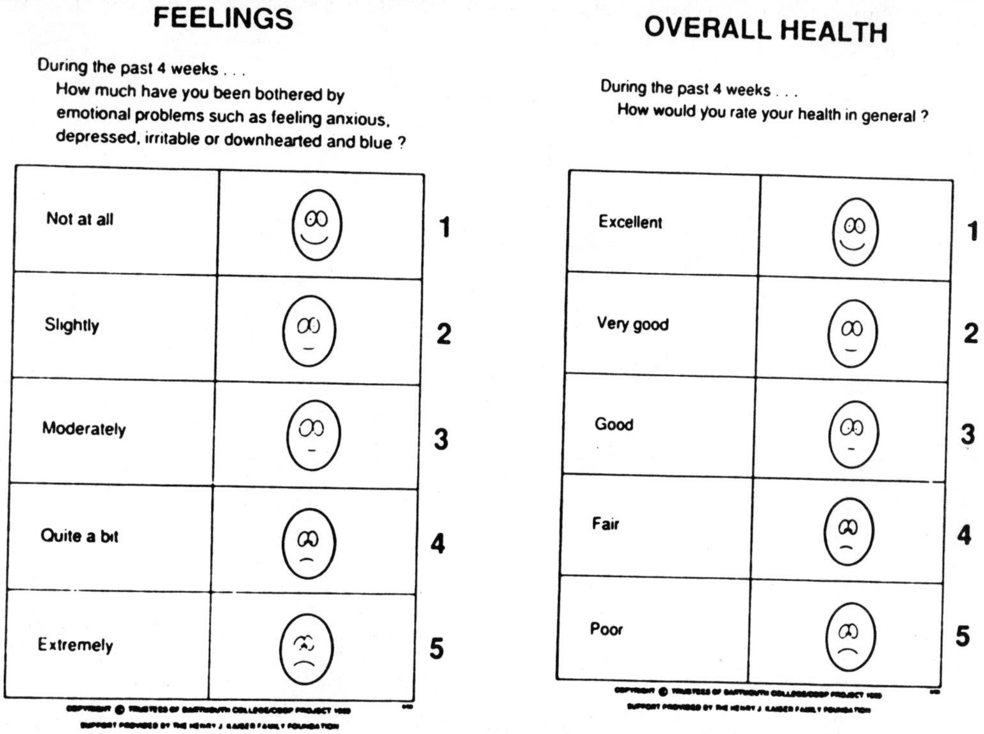

**OVERALL HEALTH**

During the past 4 weeks . . . .
How would you rate your health in general ?

| Excellent | | 1 |
| Very good | | 2 |
| Good | | 3 |
| Fair | | 4 |
| Poor | | 5 |

**FEELINGS**

During the past 4 weeks . . . .
How much have you been bothered by
emotional problems such as feeling anxious,
depressed, irritable or downhearted and blue ?

| Not at all | | 1 |
| Slightly | | 2 |
| Moderately | | 3 |
| Quite a bit | | 4 |
| Extremely | | 5 |

Figure 13.1. Continued

155

## CHANGE IN HEALTH

How would you rate your overall health
now compared to 4 weeks ago ?

| | | |
|---|---|---|
| ++ ◀◀ | **1** | Much better |
| + ◀ | **2** | A little better |
| = ↕ | **3** | About the same |
| − ▶ | **4** | A little worse |
| −− ▶▶ | **5** | Much worse |

## PAIN

During the past 4 weeks . . . .
How much bodily pain have you
generally had ?

| | | |
|---|---|---|
| | **1** | No pain |
| | **2** | Very mild pain |
| | **3** | Mild pain |
| | **4** | Moderate pain |
| | **5** | Severe pain |

## SOCIAL SUPPORT

During the past 4 weeks . . . .
Was someone available to help you if you
needed and wanted help? For example if you

– felt very nervous, lonely, or blue
– got sick and had to stay in bed
– needed someone to talk to
– needed help with daily chores
– needed help just taking care of yourself

| | |
|---|---|
| Yes, as much as I wanted | 1 |
| Yes, quite a bit | 2 |
| Yes, some | 3 |
| Yes, a little | 4 |
| No, not at all | 5 |

## QUALITY OF LIFE

How have things been going for you during the past 4 weeks?

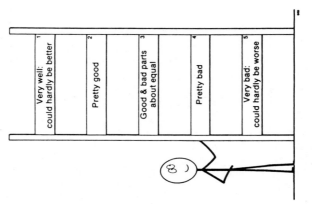

| | |
|---|---|
| Very well: could hardly be better | 1 |
| Pretty good | 2 |
| Good & bad parts about equal | 3 |
| Pretty bad | 4 |
| Very bad: could hardly be worse | 5 |

**Figure 13.2.** Continued

157

requires about 30-45 seconds to complete; most patients can complete all nine in less than 5 minutes. The answer sheet can be included in the patient's medical record and forwarded to the clinician or be part of a larger research questionnaire.

## Methods of Evaluating the COOP Chart System

The COOP charts were evaluated through their use on more than 1,400 patients sampled from four clinical settings. Each setting used different protocols to evaluate one or more aspects of the charts. Results from each setting were treated and analyzed independently (Nelson et al., 1990b).

### VARIABILITY

Analysis of a measure must determine whether the instrument is sensitive enough to detect differences between patients from diverse populations (i.e., show variability). With single-item instruments such as the COOP charts the principle of variability is very important. The distribution of responses for all nine charts is shown in Table 13.1. All showed substantial variation in scores: standard deviations ranged from 0.66 to 1.6, and the full range of scores was observed on all charts. The mean scores ranged from a low of 1.3 (Social Support) to a high of 3.2 (Overall Health). Most measures were somewhat skewed toward the Good Health end of the scale; the one most skewed was Social Support.

### RELIABILITY

Given the single-item nature of each chart, we used two forms of test-retest reliability to assess the charts:

1. *Test-retest reliability with the same method of administration* was done in several settings, with varying techniques and patient populations, with intervals ranging from 1 hour to 16 days on average in order to determine stability of the scores over time. Reliability of 0.90 or higher, of test-retest correlation, has been recommended (Nunnally, 1978).

The reliability of the charts was outstanding in the 1-hour test-retest studies. In one sample, correlation coefficients ranged from 0.93 to 0.99, and kappas were all in the excellent range (from 0.80 to 0.97). In a second sample, correlation coefficients ranged from 0.74 to 0.98, and five kappas were excellent, three were good, and one was fair. As expected, the lower socioeconomic status in the second sample was reflected in generally

**Table 13.1** Descriptive Statistics: Means and Standard Deviations of Chart Scores in Different Patient Samples

| COOP CHART | COOP (1A) | | COOP (1b) | | VA (2) | | BG (3) | | MOS (4) | |
|---|---|---|---|---|---|---|---|---|---|---|
| | Mean | S.D | Mean | S.D. | Mean | S.D. | Mean | S.D. | Mean | S.D. |
| | N=225 | | N=147 | | N=231 | | N=51 | | N=784 | |
| Physical Function | 2.8 | 1.2 | 2.6 | 1.3 | 2.5 | 1.3 | 3.1 | 1.6 | 2.41 | 1.2 |
| Emotional Status | 2.1 | 1.1 | 2.6 | 1.2 | 2.1 | 1.0 | 2.2 | 1.2 | 2.0 | 1.1 |
| Role Function | 1.9 | 1.0 | 2.2 | 1.1 | 2.4 | 1.3 | 2.0 | 1.2 | 1.7 | 1.0 |
| Social Function | 1.8 | 1.0 | 1.9 | 1.1 | 1.9 | 1.2 | 1.8 | 1.3 | 1.6 | 0.9 |
| Pain | 2.5 | 1.3 | 2.6 | 1.3 | 1.5 | 1.0 | 2.5 | 1.5 | 2.5 | 1.3 |
| Health Change | 2.5 | .99 | 2.8 | 1.0 | 2.9 | 0.8 | 2.7 | 0.9 | 3.3 | 0.8 |
| Overall Health | 2.8 | 1.0 | 3.0 | 1.0 | 3.2 | 0.9 | 2.9 | 1.2 | 2.6 | 1.0 |
| Social Support | 1.3 | .66 | 1.9 | 1.1 | 1.6 | 1.2 | 1.9 | 1.4 | 1.7 | 1.1 |
| Quality of Life | 1.8 | .87 | 2.2 | 0.9 | - | - | 2.2 | 1.0 | 2.1 | 0.8 |

(1A) New London Medical Centre Practices in New England
(1B) General COOP Practices in New England
(2) Veterans Administration Outpatient Clinic, WRJ
(3) Bowman Gray School of Medicine
(4) Medical Outcomes Study
* Chart scores range from 1-5; 5 indicates poorest health except for Health Change Chart scores, a score of 3 indicates "no change," 1 and 2 indicate improvement, and 4 and 5 indicate decline in health.

lower reliability of the charts. Thus most charts exhibit strong test-retest reliability even when used on elderly and socially disadvantaged patients.

Since the relatively short time interval (1 hour) may have resulted in inflated reliability estimates because of recall effects, reassessment in one group 2 weeks later resulted in correlation coefficients ranging from 0.42 to 0.88. Role Function had the highest correlation, Quality of Life the lowest. As expected, reliabilities were lower for most charts than they had been at 1 hour. The lower level of agreement may be due to a change in actual health status or to less opportunity for recall of one's prior ratings.

2. *Test-retest reliability with different administrators* measures the agreement with readministration by two or more examiners at a fixed time interval (e.g., the same day). The more reliable the charts, the greater the agreement expected between scores, using Pearson's product-moment correlations and kappa, where appropriate.

Consistent with accepted guidelines, kappa reliability correlations in the following ranges were given these descriptive labels: "excellent" is >.74, "good" is .60-.74, "fair" is .40-.59, and "poor" is <.40 (Fleiss, 1981).

For the interrater reliability assessment, eight of the nine correlation coefficients were 0.76 or better; one, that for Role Function, was 0.60.

Four of the charts had excellent kappas; two, good; and three, fair or poor (Nelson et al., 1990b).

## VALIDITY

How accurately do the COOP charts measure what they are designed to measure, that is, how the patients feel, function, and perceive their health? Their empirical validity was evaluated using several approaches:

*Association With Validity Indicator Variables.* We tested the relationship between the charts and selected demographic variables and health measures, using the following validity indicator variables: number of disability days, number of symptoms, level of cognitive function, amount of sleep disturbances and sleep respiratory problems, reported walking pace, energy/fatigue level, perceived resistance to illness, health outlook and health distress, satisfaction with family, family function, and reported life events. Higher levels of dysfunction as measured by the charts would be expected to be directly associated with worse levels of health status.

We calculated correlations between the COOP charts and established measures of health, perceptions of health, and other validity indicator variables for 784 chronic-disease patients. These variables were selected to represent the range of possible health and related measures from the MOS baseline patient assessment questionnaire. Almost without exception the association between the charts and the validity variables is statistically significant in the expected direction. The more subjective health measures—for example, symptoms, energy/fatigue, resistance to illness, health outlook, and health distress—tended to correlate somewhat more highly with the charts (correlations ranging from .15 to .58) than did the more objective ones— for example, disability days and walking pace (.02 to .30). Life events, family functioning, and family satisfaction have significant effects on all charts except Physical Function. Social Support was least related to other health measures; this was expected because it is least directly linked to health. Further details have been published elsewhere (Nelson et al., 1990b).

In a VA sample, correlation of the charts with selected clinical measures also reveals moderate correlations in the expected direction (Nelson et al., 1990b). Correlations of "number of symptoms" with each of the chart scores was significant, ranging from 0.25 (Health Change) to 0.51 (Overall Health). A "chronic illness" score was significantly associated with all the charts except Emotional Status and Health Change, and "number of medications" was significantly related to all except Health Change and Social Support.

*Convergent Validity: Association With Paired Measures.* Many of the charts were designed to measure areas similar but not identical to the previously validated MOS long-form measures (Nelson et al., 1990b). On the whole the correlations between paired charts and MOS measures of health in three different samples were impressive, ranging from 0.48 to 0.78, similar to intercorrelations between other health status instruments with the majority in the 0.60 to 0.70 range. In addition shared variance between the charts and the paired measures was substantial, ranging from 20% to 61% for Physical Function, 38% to 49% for Emotional Function, 35% to 42% for Role Function, and 26% to 35% for Overall Health. These relations suggest that the charts tap information similar to that measured by longer, standardized health measures and provide support for their convergent validity.

*Discriminant Validity: Multitrait-Multimethod Analysis.* The powerful multitrait-multimethod (MTMM) analysis (Campbell & Fiske, 1959; Hayashi & Hays, 1987) compared the charts to the relevant multi-item MOS measures to assess convergent and discriminant validity in 592 chronic-disease patients. The average convergent validity correlation between the different measures of the same concept was 0.60, exceeding the average off-diagonal correlation of 0.35, between different concepts measured by either the same or different methods (Nelson et al., 1990b). This result supports the generally good discriminant validity of the measures.

We compared convergent validity correlations with appropriate off-diagonal correlations (Campbell & Fiske, 1959). Different measures of the same trait tended to correlate significantly more highly with one another than did measures of different traits (96% of the heteromethod and 70% of the monomethod comparisons were statistically significant in the hypothesized direction). The Hays-Hayashi Quality Index was 0.82 (possible range negative infinity to 1.0), indicating overall generally good discriminant validity for the measures. Although the convergent and discriminant validities of most charts were quite good, two trouble spots appeared. Role and Social Function had clear discriminant validity problems, with only 50% and 42%, respectively, of monomethod comparisons being statistically significant in the hypothesized direction.

Similar findings were obtained from the MTMM analysis performed on 229 elderly patients in a VA sample (Nelson et al., 1990b).

*Known Groups Validity.* To determine whether the COOP charts were as accurate as the MOS short-form survey in detecting the impact of disease on patient functioning, we compared 20 measures of disease status and demographic variables (i.e., known diagnostic and socioeconomic groups) as independent variables, using the COOP and MOS measures as dependent variables (Nelson et al., 1990b). Dependent variables all were transformed linearly to a common 0-100 score distribution in a multiple regression analysis.

In general the presence of medically verified diseases have a measurable influence—in the expected way—on the level of the patients' health as measured by the nine charts. Our studies allowed us to compare this influence on the charts' measure with that on the MOS measures. Care must be taken, however, in interpreting the charts versus the MOS parameters, because of differences in the distributions of the two scales and different times when they were administered, allowing the possibility of interval change in patients' health status. Such change would make the charts appear less sensitive to the influence of disease.

Bearing these differences in mind, the effects observed for the charts generally mirror those observed for the MOS short-form health measures. Except for Emotional Status, the amount of explained variance was similar in corresponding chart and MOS measures (for example, the proportion of variance explained for the chart and the MOS physical function measures was 30% and 27%, respectively). In addition the predictor variables used for both the chart and MOS regressions tend to have the same sign and similar patterns of statistical significance (e.g., having an MI significantly decreases the predicted score of both measures of physical, role, and overall health). The Emotional Function difference in proportion of variance explained was substantial: $r$-squares for the chart versus the MOS measure were 0.30 and 0.52, respectively. This difference was largely attributable to the level of correlation between depressive symptoms and emotional status as defined by the charts and the MOS measures ($r$'s = 0.49 vs. 0.69; standardized betas: −0.41 vs. −0.64).

## Acceptability and Clinical Utility

If the charts are going to be both useful and used, the main consumers—clinicians and patients—must find them acceptable in routine use. How do clinicians and patients react to use of the charts: Are the charts easy to understand and answer, and enjoyable to use? Can the charts be easily integrated into routine office practice? What effect do the charts have on the management of patients? Do the charts affect the communication between the patient and clinician? Do the charts provide the clinician with new or useful information about the patient? Do the charts stimulate new management actions in the care of the patient?

Postvisit questionnaires completed by five office nurses and 225 patients showed that 89% of the patients enjoyed using the charts and that 93% reported they liked the chart illustrations. Nurses' enjoyment and patients' liking of the illustrations did not differ significantly by patients' sex, age, educational level, or marital status. According to the nurses 99% of the patients understood the charts, whereas 97% of the patients reported understanding them. This understanding did not differ by demographic variables. Debriefing interviews held with office staff from 11 practices indicated that (a) the charts are not difficult to integrate into office routine for gathering information on patients, and (b) sets of four charts took 2-3 three minutes for nurses to administer to patients.

*Providers Perspective:* Highlights of the debriefing interviews are provided in the 23 case histories (available on request from the authors). This qualitative information showed that use of the charts regularly provides important information, frequently leads to the discovery of previously unrecognized problems, at times shows better than expected functioning, and improves communication between patients and clinician. Some clinicians seemed to attribute more value to the charts than others, with ratings of chart utility being significantly different across individuals. The effect of the charts on physician-patient communication as viewed by the physician was rated as positive for 13% of patients, no effect for 85%, and negative for only 2%.

An important finding from the postvisit questionnaires completed by physicians was that for 25% of patients seen the charts led to new information. Moreover physicians reported that for 40% of this group this new information led to changes in their clinical management. This finding suggests that use of the charts may stimulate changes in what physicians know about their patients and how they treat them, which in theory could lead to subsequent improvements in health status.

*Patient's View:* The postvisit questionnaires completed by patients provided further evidence supporting the utility of the charts. Almost 9 out of 10 reported that the information they had provided on the charts was important for their doctors to know. More than three fourths (76%) indicated that the charts influenced their communication with the doctor, and 85% indicated that the charts affected management actions. Most patients rated the charts to be useful: 10%, excellent; 21%, very good; 43%, good; 23%, fair; and only 3%, poor. Patient ratings were unrelated to most demographic variables. The effect of the charts on communication, however, was related to sex: 86% of male patients versus 69% of females reported that the charts influenced their communication with their physicians.

## DISCUSSION

*Summary, and Implications for Clinical Practice.* We set out to develop a set of measures that could be used in busy office practices to screen and monitor patient functioning. First, on the positive side we found that the charts are reliable, generating reproducible results when administered properly. (Although the reliability of self-administration was not tested, it probably would yield similar results). Second, we found that the charts produce valid information. They are strongly associated with related measures that have undergone validation. They are correlated with health and clinical status in the expected manner. Perhaps most importantly, they detect dysfunction associated with major chronic diseases almost as well as other validated multi-item measures. Third, we learned that the "consumers" involved—physicians, office nurses, and patients—all indicated that the charts can be beneficial and are not difficult to use, understand, or interpret. Most patients enjoyed using the charts and believed the charts measured important aspects of health. Fourth, with respect to clinical utility, physicians who used the charts indicated that they generated new information on about one out of four patients. The more than 20 case studies we collected provide further evidence supporting this clinical utility.

On the negative side are occasions when the charts may have a deleterious effect on physician-patient communication. This is a very infrequent event—occurring roughly 2% of the time according to physicians—but it still merits further thought and a note of caution. Second, some of the charts probably could be improved. For example, the MTMM results, while mostly showing good convergent and discriminant validity, showed a good deal of "overlap" between the chart measures of physical function and role function, as well as for the MOS short-form measures of the same dimensions. Third, some physicians seemed to attribute more value to the charts than others. For example, ratings of clinical utility were significantly different across individual clinicians. Fourth, even though the charts do not take long to use, if they are administered by the nurse, medical assistant, or physician, as opposed to being self-administered, a substantial "cost-effectiveness" trade-off would always exist. Consequently we need to determine which charts are most useful for what kinds of patients and at what interval of time.

*Limitations and Future Directions.* Much work has been done to assess the reliability, validity, acceptability, and clinical utility of the charts, but further work is needed. Concerning reliability it would be useful to (a) better determine how reliability varies as a function of clinician, patient, and setting;

(b) conduct more refined studies involving various test-retest time periods to clarify the importance of the recall factor; and (c) establish the reliability of self-administration vis-à-vis clinician-administration.

Concerning validity, we need to (a) learn more about the ability of the charts to detect actual changes occurring within the individual patient's level of function over time and those linked to known changes in treatment or natural history; (b) obtain better discrimination between different dimensions of health and thereby improve our ability to differentiate role function from physical function; (c) learn how to calibrate the levels of the chart scores to clinically relevant events (such as the effect of having an MI or experiencing depression); and (d) determine how to assign weighted values to each of the five levels of each respective chart to reflect the magnitude of the intervals between the levels in addition to their clear rank order.

Although the charts have shown good acceptability in many diverse settings, we know little about (a) how much the charts' illustrations enhance (or detract from) their acceptability and measurement properties, and (b) how easy it would be to disseminate the charts more widely to medical practices around the world. The ultimate test of the charts' value of course has to do with their clinical utility and their utility in practice-based research. Will regular medical practitioners really use them routinely? If they are used, what new information is produced and on what types of patients? How frequently does this new information actually effect a change in the management plan? Finally how frequently do certain types of patients benefit in terms of measurable gains in function (or at least less rapid deterioration) than would otherwise be the case?

Do the charts need to be linked, as we think they do, to more in-depth yet practical assessment tools that physicians can use to work up patients who have problems? Would physicians benefit from education and training in such topics as a functional approach to patient care and/or how to evaluate and manage patient function? Although much work lies ahead, the charts appear to be reliable, valid, and acceptable. Their routine use with certain types of patients could make an important contribution to better care.

# References

Bergner, M., Bobbit, R. A., Carter, W. B., Kressel, S., Pollard, W. E., Gilson, B. S., & Morris J. R. (1976). The sickness impact profile: Conceptual formulation and methodology for the development of a health status measure. *International Journal of Health Services, 6,* 393.

Campbell, D. T., & Fiske, D. W. (1959). Convergent and discriminant validation by the multitrait-y matrix. *Psychological Bulletin, 56,* 81-105.

Criteria Committee of the New York Heart Association, Inc. (1964). *Diseases of the heart and blood vessels: Nomenclature and criteria for diagnosis of diseases of the heart and great vessels* (6th ed.). Boston: Little, Brown.

Fleiss, J. L. (1981). *Statistical methods for rates and proportions.* New York: John Wiley.

Goldman, L., Hashimoto, B., Cook, E. F., & Loscalzo, A. (1981). Comparative reproducibility and validity of systems for assessing cardiovascular functional class: Advantages of a new specific activity scale. *Circulation, 64*(6), 1277-1334.

Hayashi, T., & Hays, R. D. (1987). A microcomputer program for analyzing multitrait-multimethod matrices: Behavior research methods. *Instruments and Computers, 19,* 345.

Hunt, S. M., McEwen, J., & McKennan, S. P. (1985). Measuring health status: A tool for clinicians and epidemiologists. *Journal of the Royal College of General Practitioners, 35,* 185-188.

Katz, S., Ford, A. B., Moskowitz, R. W., Jackson, B. A., & Jaffe, M. W. (1963). Studies of illness in the aged. The index of ADL: A standardized measure of biological and psychosocial function. *Journal of the American Medical Association, 185,* 914-919.

McDowell, I., & Newell, C. (1987). *Measuring health: A guide to rating scales and questionnaires.* New York: Oxford University Press.

Nelson, E., Conger, B., Douglass, R., Gephart, D., Kirk, J., Page, R., Clark, A., Johnson, K., Stone, D., Wasson, J., & Zubkoff, M. (1983). Functional health status level of primary care patients. *Journal of the American Medical Association, 249*(24), 3331-3338.

Nelson, E. C., Landgraf, J. M., Hays, R. D., Kirk, J. W., Wasson, J. H., Keller, A., & Zubkoff, M. (1987). *The COOP function charts: A system to assess functional health status in physicians' offices.* Final report to Henry J. Kaiser Family Foundation. Hanover, NH: Dartmouth Medical School.

Nelson, E. C., Landgraf, J. M., Hays, R. D., Kirk, J. W., Wasson, J. H., Keller, A., & Zubkoff, M. (1990b). The COOP function charts: A system to measure patient function in physicians' offices. In M. Lipkin, Jr. (Ed.), *Frontiers of primary care: Functional status measurement in primary care* (pp.97-131). Stony Brook, NY: Springer-Verlag.

Nelson, E. C., Landgraf, J. M., Hays, R. D., Wasson, J. H., & Kirk, J. W. (1990a). The functional status of patients: How can it be measured in physicians' offices? *Medical Care, 28*(12), 1111-1126.

Nelson, E. C., Wasson, J. H., & Kirk, J. W. (1987). Assessment of function in routine clinical practice: Description of the COOP chart method and preliminary findings. *Journal of Chronic Disease, 50*(S1), 55S.

Nunnally, C. (1978). *Psychometric theory* (2nd ed.). New York: McGraw-Hill.

Parkerson, G. R., Jr., Gehlback, S. H., Wagner, E. G., James, S. A., Clapp, N. E., & Muhlbaier, L. H. (1981). The Duke-UNC health profile: An adult health status instrument for primary care. *Medical Care, 19,* 806-828.

Sackett, D., Chambers, L., MacPherson, A. S., Goldsmith, C. H., & Macauley, R. G. (1977). The development and application of indices of health: General methods and a summary of results. *American Journal of Public Health, 67,* 423-427.

Ware, J. E., Jr. (1987). Standards for validating health measures: Definition and content. *Journal of Chronic Disease, 40,* 473-480.

Ware, J. E., Brook, R. H., Davies-Avery, A., Williams, K. N., & Stewart, A. L. (1980). *Conceptualization and measurement of health for adults in the health insurance study: Vol. I. Model of health and methodology* (R-1987/1-HEW). Santa Monica: RAND Corp.

Ware, J. E., Johnston, S. A., Davies-Avery, A., & Brook, R. H. (1979). *Conceptualization and measurement of health for adults in the health insurance study: Vol. III. Mental health* (R-1987/3-HEW). Santa Monica: RAND Corp.

# PART FOUR

# TOOLS FOR DATA COLLECTION

# 14 The Medical Record as a Source of Information for Research

RICHARD A. MacLACHLAN
BRIAN HENNEN

## Introduction

Chart review has been described as "the bridge between the concepts of traditional research and modern scholarship—for the discipline and for the individual" ("Research, Audit," 1985, p. 191). It follows the same rules as other forms of research, which are to (a) ask a good question, (b) identify a single answerable part of the question, (c) ensure that the data collected will reliably answer the question, and (d) respond to what is found.

A number of types of studies exist for which chart reviews can be useful, as follows:

*Quality Improvement.* Chart review can be the basis for a professional quality improvement program. It is important for a self-regulating profession to be able to define standards and to have a mechanism that is effective in identifying deficiencies specifically enough to facilitate response and improvement. In medical practice this will often involve a retrospective review of charts but can equally well include prospective data gathering with encounter forms that summarize individual patient visits (Lamberts, 1991).

*"What's Happening in My Practice?"* Physicians need a mechanism to "take the pulse" of their practices. This mechanism might include such areas as hypertension screening rates, migration of patients, patient satisfaction, or the proportion of elderly patients seen at home in a year. Physicians need to be able to respond to issues of concern to their practice populations and to identify barriers to their optimal care and health.

169

*Continuing Medical Education.*  Chart review is an effective method of directing continuing medical education, which is concerned with both the acquisition of knowledge and its application. Learning theorists report that physicians prefer to be self-directed learners, to use a problem-oriented patient-centered approach, and to be able to apply their new knowledge and skills immediately (Putnam, 1987).

McWhinney (1981a) has described the necessary conditions for effective learning from day-to-day experience in one's own practice. These are:

1. Physicians must know about their own experience, including the outcomes of their actions in both the long and the short term.
2. Standards should exist against which to measure performance.
3. Physicians must have the capacity to accept criticism and the ability to make changes to their method of practice.

Chart reviews encourage physicians to assimilate information from many sources, such as literature, consultants, and previous experience, in order to develop standards of care that are applicable to their practice settings.

*Exploring Unanswered Questions.*  This is where chart reviews clearly cross into the domain of research. Research has been described as "organized curiosity" (Eimerl, 1960). Chart reviews allow physicians to explore such questions as, "Could I have made the diagnosis earlier?" (e.g., cancer or depression) or "What happens to patients with this symptom over time?" (e.g., backache or migraine). To answer such questions as these can be very rewarding. Chart review and its related research activities allow one to appraise critically one's own practice and to add to both personal and collective knowledge of disease and health.

## Focus on the Medical Record

Family doctors have been assessing their practices in various ways. The E book of the British Royal College of General Practitioners has been the basis for an Age/Sex Register and diagnostic frequency data for a number of years (McWhinney, 1981b). That kind of format is now available in various computer programs using the ICHPPC System (International Classification of Health Problems in Primary Care, 1983) or more recently the ICPC (International Classification of Primary Care, Chapter 4 in this volume; and Lamberts & Wood, 1987). In the late 1930s Will Pickles, in his classic book *The Epidemiology of Country Practice*, demonstrated how an individual practitioner, by keeping careful records, could assess certain aspects of his or her practice (Pickles, 1972).

Beginning in the late 1960s Donabedian (1980), Brook and Appel, (1973), Kessner, Kalk, and Singer (1973), and Sibley et al. (1975) were among those who developed the concept of tracer (or indicator) conditions to be used in ambulatory care as a means of practice audit. A *tracer condition* is defined as "a condition that is known to have a functional impact on patients, is relatively well-defined and easy to diagnose, occurs frequently enough to allow a reasonable sample size from the practice population under study, and is one for which the natural history is felt to be alterable by medical intervention." In addition it is one for which the management is well defined for at least one of the diagnostic or rehabilitation aspects of care, and the effects of nonmedical factors on it are understood.

## HOW TO SAMPLE CHARTS

Ideally, chart sampling should be done randomly. Efficiency demands, however, that representative charts that are richest in information be selected. Borgiel et al. (1989), in assessing individual doctor's performances, used random selection of charts for review but discarded those in which more than one third of the patient's encounters had been with providers other than the doctor under review. One pediatrician, in reviewing perinatal hospital records in any one unit, has reported selecting 10 records at random and 10 from high-risk patients (Dr. G. Chance, personal communication, June 1990). For everyday self-assessment activities in practice settings, blindness in selection is probably far less important than getting on with the process of regular review.

## HOW MANY CHARTS SHOULD BE REVIEWED?

Some authors have put forth cautious recommendations for the number of visit records to be reviewed in a quality improvement program. Borgiel et al. (1989) developed criteria for 182 tracer conditions. When they subsequently reviewed 25 records per physician, they found that 90.6% of the charts reviewed contained at least one of these conditions. Putnam (1987), using a record audit as a means for directing Continuing Medical Education, recommended 15-30 cases for each tracer condition being assessed. In the authors' experience with over 20 diagnosis-related chart reviews with residents, we have used 30-35 charts per review of one condition. The College of Physicians and Surgeons of Ontario surveyors reviewed 20-25 randomly selected charts (McAuley et al., 1990). Stewart (1984), in her studies of doctor-patient relationships, determined that when audio transcripts, rich in detail, were used, 10 consultations were sufficient.

## ABSTRACTION OF DATA

How should the information extracted from the chart be recorded, and who should do the extraction? For efficiency and uniformity it is wise to design a data extraction sheet that allows one to record quickly the information desired and that has some means of being linked to the record while preserving confidentiality. If the sheet can be organized so that trained nonmedical staff can do the extraction, the review will be less demanding of physician time. Audits of hospital charts are frequently done by staff of the medical records department.

Training others as abstractors was accomplished successfully by the authors while teaching audit to residents. A secretary who participated with the residents in the development of the criteria and of the abstract worksheets became a very efficient record assessor and was able to summarize the data very quickly in tabular form. Her involvement not only gave her a sense of the meaning intended but helped us develop criteria in language that was clear and easily applied by such abstractors. Borgiel et al. (1989) found inter-rater reliability between physician and nurse auditors to be .84. This group also held workshops to prepare abstractors to apply predetermined criteria.

## VALIDITY AND COMPLETENESS OF RECORDS

The most controversial methodological issue is related to the validity of the medical record as a reflection of practice behavior. Romm and Putnam (1981), in a comparison of records with verbatim transcripts of outpatient visits, determined that 59% of units of information that were present in the transcripts were also found in the records. The most frequently recorded was chief complaint (92%); next was information related to the present illness (71%); and other items in the medical history were recorded in only 29% of cases reviewed. The working rule of record-based reviews must be "If it isn't written down, it didn't happen," and this is a fundamental basis for such reviews.

Stewart's (1975) studies of doctor-patient relationships involved transcripts of office consultations by general practitioners. Symptom considerations were reasonably reflected in their records, but patient concerns and functional status were not.

The College of Physicians and Surgeons of Ontario has determined statistical significance in the relation between deficient records and unsatisfactory care. The sensitivity of such records in identifying unsatisfactory care was 93%; and the specificity, 88% (McAuley et al., 1990).

## EXAMPLES OF CHART REVIEW

The College of Family Physicians of Canada (Borgiel et al., 1985) measured the quality assessment of care in general practice using four methods: a questionnaire on the organizational features of the practice (facilities, equipment, staff, hours, procedures); an inspection of chart format; the investigation of preventive procedures; and the use of tracer conditions. In 1985 the Royal College of General Practice (Baker, 1988) determined similar targets for review and identified as likely sources of information a practice profile (questionnaire); direct observation; discussion with staff; inspection of registers, indices, and records; a review of videotape visits and records; and an interview with the doctor.

In 1989 Borgiel et al. reported the results of their study of 120 randomly selected family physicians in Ontario. The study compared four groups of family physicians and focused on determining whether residency training made a difference in practice as measured by the study group's practice assessment program. The practices were assessed against predetermined criteria for charting, procedures in periodic health examination, quality of medical care (as measured by tracer conditions), and the use of indicator drugs. This study provided an opportunity to refine a quality assessment tool and its application using an on-site computer data entry format. The method has since been used by the College of Family Physicians of Canada to do practice assessments on practice-eligible (as opposed to residency-trained) candidates for the certification examination.

The College of Physicians and Surgeons of Ontario, a provincial licensing body, has conducted practice quality assessment reviews for 10 years (McAuley et al., 1990). It has worked cooperatively with a program of physicians' skills improvement called the Physician Enhancement Program to establish a full program including both competence review and targeted education (Davis et al., 1990).

## Outcomes

How do such reviews improve physician performance and patient care? First, it is a stimulating learning exercise to participate in discussions about what is important, what standards are acceptable, and what justifications exist for standards. Second, the in-house reviews by the authors in the Dalhousie Family Medicine Teaching Practice over 3 years

**Table 14.1** Dalhousie Department of Family Medicine Repeat Audits of Six Tracer Conditions

| TRACER CONDITION | TIME BETWEEN AUDITS (MOS.) | % CHANGE IN PROPORTION OF +VE CRITERIA RECORDED | CHI SQUARE (P) |
|---|---|---|---|
| MENOPAUSE | 15 | +20% | 14.0 (.001) |
| DIABETES | 11 | +45% | 120.9 (.001) |
| SINUSITIS | 12 | +17% | 27.4 (.001) |
| POST PARTUM CARE | 11 | + 3% | 5.4 (.05) |
| ACUTE U.T.I. | 15 | +20% | 36.6 (.001) |
| VAGINITIS | 12 | +20% | 63.9 (.001) |

showed a difference in care as recorded by seven teaching practices. During that time 6 of 21 audit topics were repeated and showed improvement in the number of standardized criteria to be met (Table 14.1). Third, Dickie and Bass (1980), in a small study involving teaching practices, determined that a self-administered audit had more impact on changing behavior than did an externally imposed one, which in turn had more effect than no audit alone. Finally, the external review process of the College of Physicians and Surgeons of Ontario has been able to demonstrate improved performance in the majority of instances in which peer assessment of practice using peer review of records identified performance deficiencies (McAuley et al., 1990).

## Conclusions

The assurance of quality medical care is increasingly important to patients, providers, planners, and insurers. Physicians can use chart review as a basis for continual exploration of symptoms and improvement in the care provided. Ryle's words of 1936 are apt today: "There is no disease of which a fuller or additional description does not remain to be written; there is no symptom as yet adequately explored" (Ryle, 1936, p. 22).

# References

Baker, R. (1988). *Practice assessment and quality of care*. (Occasional Paper 39) London: Royal College of General Practitioners.

Borgiel, A. E. M., Williams, J. I., Anderson, G. M., Bass, M. J., Dunn, E. V., Lamont, C. T., Spasoff, R. A., & Rice, D. I. (1985). Assessing the quality of care in family physicians' practices. *Canadian Family Physician, 31*, 833-862.

Borgiel, A. E. M., Williams, J. I., Bass, M. J., Dunn, E. V., Eversen, M. K., Lamont, C. T., MacDonald, P. J., McCoy, J. M., & Spasoff, R. A. (1989). Quality of care in family practice: Does residency training make a difference? *Canadian Medical Association Journal, 140*, 1035-1042.

Brook, R. H., & Appel, F. A. (1973). Quality-of-care assessment: Choosing a method for peer review. *New England Journal of Medicine, 228*, 1323-1329.

Davis, D. A., Norman, G. R., Painvin, A., Lindsay, E., Ragbeer, M. S., & Rath, D. (1990). Attempting to ensure physician competence. *Journal of the American Medical Association, 263*, 2041-2042.

Dickie, G. L., & Bass, M. J. (1980). Improving problem-oriented medical records through self-audit. *Journal of Family Practice, 10*(3), 498-490.

Donabedian, A. (1980). *The definition of quality and approaches to its assessment*. Ann Arbor, MI: Health Administration Press.

Eimerl, T. S. (1960). Organized curiosity. *Journal of the College of General Practitioners, 3*, 246-252.

Froom, J. (1983). *ICHPPC-2-Defined (International Classification of Health Problems in Primary Care)*. (1983). Prepared by the Classification Committee of WONCA (World Organization of National Colleges, Academies, and Academic Associations of General Practitioners/Family Physicians) in collaboration with the World Health Organization. Oxford, UK: Oxford University Press.

Kessner, D. M., Kalk, C. E., & Singer, J. (1973). Assessing health quality: The cases for tracers. *New England Journal of Medicine, 288*, 189-193.

Lamberts, H. (1991). Episode-oriented epidemiology in family practice: The practical use of the international classification of primary care as illustrated in patients with headache. In P. Norton, M. Steward, F. Tudiver, et al. (Eds.), *Primary Care Research* (pp. 40-72). Newbury Park, CA: Sage.

Lamberts, H., & Wood, M. (Eds.). (1987). *ICPC international classification of primary care*. Oxford, UK: Oxford University Press.

McAuley, R. G., Paul, W. M., Morrison, G. H., et al. (1990). Five-year results of the peer assessment program of the College of Physicians and Surgeons of Ontario. *Canadian Medical Association Journal, 143*(2), 1193-1199.

McWhinney, I. R. (1981a). Continuing self-education. In I. R. McWhinney (Ed.), *An introduction to family medicine*. New York: Oxford University Press.

McWhinney, I. R. (1981b). *An introduction to family medicine*. New York: Oxford University Press.

Pickles, W. N. (1972). *Epidemiology in country practice*. Torquay, Devon, U.K.: Devonshire Press.

Putnum, R. W. (1987). Patient care appraisal: Evaluating performance. In Shires, D. B., Hennen, B. K., & Rice, D. L. (Eds.), *Family Medicine: A guidebook for practitioners of the art* (pp. 493-498). New York: McGraw-Hill.

Research, audit and scholarship—nuisance or necessity? (1985) [Editorial]. *Family Practice, 2*, 191-192.

Romm, F. J., & Putnam, S. M. (1981). The validity of the medical record. *Medical Care, 19*(3), 310-315.

Ryle, J. (1936). *The natural history of disease.* London: Oxford University Press.

Sibley, J. C., Spitzer, W. O., Rudrick, K. V., Bell, J. D., Bethune, R. D., Sackett, D. L., & Wright, K. (1975). Quality of care appraisal in primary care: A quantitative method. *Annals of Internal Medicine, 83,* 46-53.

Stewart, M. A. (1975). *A study of the holistic approach in primary care.* Unpublished doctoral dissertation, The University of Western Ontario, London, Ontario.

Stewart, M. A. (1984). What is a successful doctor-patient interview—A study of interactions and outcomes. *Social Science and Medicine, 19,* 167-175.

# 15 Designing Focus Group Research

DAVID L. MORGAN

After languishing for more than 30 years, group interviews in general and focus groups in particular are once again receiving attention from behavioral science researchers. Recent work has emphasized their strengths as both a self-contained means of gathering qualitative data and as a component of triangulated research designs involving other methods. Focus groups clearly have the potential to become one of the principal means of gathering qualitative data, with applications ranging from theory testing to program evaluation.

This chapter will begin by presenting a series of examples illustrating potential uses of focus groups by researchers in the field of primary care, as they are the major audience for this volume. The bulk of the chapter will, however, concentrate on a set of research design issues that should be of interest to focus group researchers in any field. The central tasks in that section are to outline the decisions necessary to design research using focus groups and to provide some guidelines on the factors that influence these decisions in specific cases. The final section of the chapter will expand on these relatively narrow guidelines to consider a broader, more flexible approach for designing research with focus groups.

## Applications of Focus Groups to Primary Care

The rationale for introducing focus groups through examples is that several good book-length treatments on this subject have been published. Some of these books demonstrate the long-standing interest in this technique within the field of marketing (Goldman & McDonald, 1987;

Greenbaum, 1987), while others reflect its more recent adaptation to the behavioral sciences (Krueger, 1988; Morgan, 1988).

Epidemiology is one area in which primary care researchers have used focus groups, especially with regard to perceptions of risk factors and risk-related behaviors. For example, Joseph et al. (1984) used focus groups to explore the ways that gay men coped with the threat of AIDS. In their first set of groups they kept the topics broad and exploratory; they used this information to organize the discussion in later groups around more specific topics. The primary purpose of their focus groups was to generate items for a subsequent survey on gay men's response to the AIDS epidemic.

Another purpose of focus groups is gaining contact with participants' perspectives, especially when the researchers' own experiences and feelings are different from those of the target population. This is illustrated in another epidemiological study on AIDS by Flaskerud and Rush (1989). Their goal was to examine how urban black women understood the causes, effects, and treatment of AIDS. By beginning with a discussion of beliefs about the causes and treatment of illness in general and then extending this discussion to the specific topic of AIDS, the investigators were able to show how this newer illness was incorporated into existing heath beliefs and practices.

Another area in which focus groups have been applied to health care issues is the study of doctor-patient relationships. Taylor (1989) examined the gatekeeping role associated with cost containment in health maintenance organizations. He found that the primary care physicians who participated in his focus groups reported considerable conflict with their patients due to denying the latters' requests for diagnostic procedures, choosing less effective but inexpensive treatments, restricting the number of referrals made to specialists within the plan, and denying services that were not available under the plan. Coping mechanisms that the doctors developed included spending time on education so that new patients knew what was not covered in the plan, using delaying tactics so that patients would drop requests for expensive procedures, shifting blame so that patients would see others as responsible, and simply letting the plan pay so that others would bear the burden of cost containment.

A different set of issues in doctor-patient relationships is illustrated in my own work (Morgan & Spanish, 1985) on laypersons' perceptions of heart attack risk factors. By asking people who had not had any history of coronary illness to discuss their views of who has heart attacks and why, we found that they emphasized risk factors that were subject to personal control, such as stress, exercise, and diet, but paid little attention to such factors as diabetes and family history that did not fit with a model of individual responsibility.

Health education is another area in which focus groups have been productive. Basch (1987) provides an extended review of research using focus groups in this area. For example, in a study on high blood pressure media campaigns, focus groups shed light on both the effectiveness of past messages and the possible topics for future communications. In a study of consumers' utilization of health services, the researchers compared discussions from separate groups of current users, potential users, and providers of the service. A study of sexually active teenagers produced results on their knowledge about and use of contraceptives, as well as recommendations about how to overcome obstacles to contraception. Finally Basch's own work on traffic safety issues with young drivers used separate groups for males and females to clarify issues related to fears about seatbelts, sources of changes in driving behavior, concern for others as an influence on driving, and social differences in the way young people have learned to drive.

As the studies reviewed by Basch demonstrate, focus groups can be useful in both the early, exploratory phases of research on health education and in later assessments of the effectiveness of programs and interventions. An example of an exploratory use comes from a study by Howland et al. (1989) on the underutilization of bicycle helmets among fourth, fifth, and sixth graders. Based on their discovery that the students approved of using helmets but feared being laughed at by their peers, the authors made several recommendations for designing programs to increase helmet use. An example of work with an ongoing program comes from Krueger's evaluation (1988) of a nutrition program aimed at increasing the use of locally grown vegetables in Hawaii. The finding that one component of the original program (demonstrating the actual preparation of the food and providing samples) was much more effective than two other activities (distributing recipes and placing nutritional information posters in supermarkets) led to a redesign of the program. These two examples demonstrate the opportunities for focus groups in applications related to health education.

Issues in family stress provide a final set of examples that apply focus groups to primary care. In my research with recent widows (Morgan, 1989a), the goal was to investigate findings from previous research in which contact with family members was less supportive than contacts with nonfamily. These discussions revealed that widows were more likely to experience obligations in dealing with family than in dealing with friends, that is, the providing as well as receiving of support. In addition contact was continued with family members even in the face of conflict, in contrast to the flexibility of nonfamily relations. These results strongly suggest that widows treat issues of support and conflict very differently, depending on whether they occur inside or outside the family.

A second example research in the area of family stress comes from Alzheimer's caregivers (Morgan, 1989b; 1990). Of interest here are the differences between spouses and adult children as caregivers. Caregiving for a spouse with Alzheimer's disease evolves out of a lifelong relationship to the partner; in contrast, for a daughter or son, assuming primary responsibility for a cognitively impaired parent often is an abrupt change in the relationship. Focus groups can be an effective way of comparing the experiences of different population subgroups, thereby providing insights into the appropriateness of highly generalized models.

As the examples in this section illustrate, focus groups are a very general research technique with a wide range of possible uses. They can serve as both precursors and follow-ups to other, primary research methods, or they can be a self-sufficient source of data. In some instances they will be entirely exploratory, while in others they will provide verification for prior theorizing. Likewise they sometimes serve a highly applied function, such as program evaluation, and at other times they play a pure research role, such as hypothesis generation. This breadth of applications places a premium on the effective design of research with focus groups, and that is the topic for the remainder of this chapter.

## Decision-Based Designs
## in Focus Groups

The remainder of this chapter will explore several basic design decisions that must be made in doing focus group research. Research design at this level of generality means making choices among a set of reasonably well-defined options in order to match a general technique to a specific research question. For any research method, a specific set of research design choices must be made, either implicitly or explicitly, and the chief task is to make these choices in a way that will provide the best answer to one's research question.

To move focus groups away from implicit rules of thumb and toward explicit research design choices, it is first necessary to note that the existing rules of thumb do in fact encompass the major design dimensions that apply to focus groups. The point here is not that these rules ignore design issues; instead, the problem is that they deal with these issues by imposing unquestioned standards instead of conscious choices. Fortunately a relative consensus exists about both the major design issues in focus groups and the rules of thumb for resolving these issues (Basch, 1987; Frey & Fontana, 1991; Morgan, 1988). In general it is thought that groups should be highly structured, groups should have 6 to 10 people who are homogeneous strangers, and four to six groups should be used.

The rules of thumb provide a starting point for making decisions about the kinds of focus groups that are most appropriate for a project. In essence these rules represent the choices that one would make if no particular choices were necessary. The fact that a typical form exists for focus groups can be quite useful, especially for those who are new to the field and need some point of reference. Students typically ask such questions as, How many groups should I have? or What happens if the people I want to interview already know each other? Having a central tendency provides a basis for assessing what it means to depart from the standard form. For example, by questioning the supposed advantages of using strangers, one can arrive at a list of issues that must be dealt with in conducting groups with acquaintances. Thus the central theme that runs throughout this approach to designing focus group research is, When is a departure from the general form of focus groups useful or even necessary for pursuing a specific research question?

This next section does, however, require a disclaimer. What follows is not an authoritative review of the issues underlying design decisions—that will be possible only when our knowledge about these decisions is based on the outcomes of rigorous methodological experimentation. While important precedents exist in this regard (e.g., Fern, 1982), most of the information that is currently available comes from the cumulative experience of past researchers. This presentation is thus best seen as preliminary: working toward a summary of best practices, but with the full recognition that the bases for these practices are relatively untested.

## How Structured Should the Group Be?

The above question appears first on the list because it is often the issue that must be considered first. The reason is that a great many other decisions depend on the amount of structure in the group: For example, relatively fewer groups are needed when the degree of structure is high, because the moderator can assure that each group will be as productive as possible. In addition the decision about the amount of structure is crucial because it affects the very nature of the data and thus every aspect of the research, including the analysis. Because of the central importance of this design dimension, it will receive a longer discussion than the others.

**Table 15.1** Design Alternatives for Group Structure

| DEGREE OF STRUCTURE | | |
|---|---|---|
| QUESTIONS | GROUP DYNAMICS | TYPE OF GROUP |
| High | High | Tightly Structured |
| High | Low | Phenomenological |
| Low | High | Exploratory |
| Low | Low | Loosely Structured |

In making decisions about the amount of structure to be imposed on the group, it is necessary to distinguish between two aspects of the moderator's role. The unavoidable role that a moderator performs is to ask questions of the group, and a group will be more structured to the extent that the moderator has a predetermined list of questions to be asked in a given order in each group. The second and more flexible role that a moderator performs is to manage the course of the group discussion. A group will be more structured to the extent that the moderator controls the group dynamics by determining who speaks and how much each person can say. (Frey and Fontana [1991] refer to this as a directive or nondirective role for the interviewer.) Selecting the appropriate design requires an understanding of what it means for a group to be more structured or less structured in both regards and of how these two decisions affect the data that are available for answering research questions.

One way of addressing the issue of how group structure affects data is through a distinction made by Calder (1977), comparing phenomenological approaches and exploratory approaches to focus groups (see also Basch, 1987). Phenomenological approaches emphasize learning the participants' perspectives on the focal topic; examples would include collecting accounts of participants' experiences in a given domain or getting reactions to existing research instruments. Exploratory approaches, as the name implies, are used when the primary goal is to discover more about a subject than is currently known; examples would include probing the bases for participants' preferences among a set of alternatives or generating hypotheses for future research. The argument here is that these two approaches emphasize different aspects of group structure, as summarized in Table 15.1.

According to the prevailing rule of thumb, tightly structured groups are the norm, with moderators controlling both the questions and the group dynamics. This approach is entirely appropriate when one knows what the important questions are and has a clear sense of what one wants to learn about these questions. In this case a well-trained moderator can get the maximum amount of information from the group in the most efficient fashion. These groups are also easier to analyze, as they all follow the same structure with only a minimum of detours or irrelevant discussion. When relatively little time is available for analysis, one's design decisions may put a premium on structure in the gathering of the data.

A tightly structured design is less appropriate when the goal is to encounter new perspectives on the research topics, as structure confines the information about these topics to the answers to predetermined questions. For example, a set of questions that is designed to narrow in on a specific set of issues cannot uncover whether participants are in fact more concerned with other issues. This design is also less appropriate when the goal is to get participants' spontaneous impressions, as the group dynamics surrounding the responses to the questions are controlled by the moderator. For example, a response that has been heard frequently in previous groups may be cut off, regardless of the inherent uncertainty about how this new group would have reacted to this viewpoint. One thus needs to be certain of one's goals: If no priority is put on experiencing the phenomenology of participants' perspectives, and if it is not important to explore all avenues of participants' thinking, then tightly structured groups offer many advantages.

The phenomenological approach described by Calder (1977) represents a design decision in which the researcher still determines the questions to be asked but exercises less control over the interaction within the groups. Margaret Spanish and I used this approach in our research on the perception of heart attack risk factors (Morgan & Spanish, 1985), in which we wished to hear the participants' perspectives without imposing our own point of view. We asked participants first to tell us stories about people they knew who had had heart attacks and then to use these stories to discuss who has heart attacks and why. We termed these groups "self-managed" to reflect the fact that the participants controlled their own discussions. Because of the more flexible interaction in self-managed groups and the tendency for the same material to be repeated from group to group, this approach will be less efficient than having a moderator control the flow of discussion. In return, however, one gets a more accurate assessment of the frequency with which given ideas and responses appear. The key advantage of phenomenological groups is that one can be relatively sure that one is getting the participants' own responses to the questions at hand.

Self-managed groups are not, however, unfocused groups. To maintain a focus on the chosen questions, it is important to give the participants instructions about how they can do their self-management tasks and for a moderator to remain present even if he or she is not sitting at the same table. The major dangers are that the discussion in a group will wander far afield or that some participants will dominate the discussion at the expense of others. These particular problems can be minimized through appropriate instructions to the participants (cf. Morgan, 1988), but they cannot be eliminated. In addition it should be obvious that this approach can lead to relatively rambling discussions, so it is often useful to ask fewer questions, given the time available. This approach is thus particularly appropriate when the goal is to produce more detailed information about a limited set of topics. It should also be obvious that the analysis of these groups will be complicated by the lack of structure in their interaction.

Exploratory groups are fundamentally even less structured than phenomenological groups, as the set of questions pursued will vary from group to group. This does not mean, however, that the discussions will be chaotic. One needs a clear sense of what the research is about in order to explore participants' ideas effectively. Given well-specified goals, it is the moderator's job to direct the groups in ways that probe the full range of participants' thoughts about the topic. Thus the emphasis is on the moderator's control of the discussion itself; the freedom to create questions is an essential element of this control. For example, if a new idea is raised, the moderator can probe the group extensively to find out whether this idea has unexplored implications or whether it is just a relatively deviant point of view.

The kind of structure imposed on the discussion in exploratory groups differs from that used in tightly structured groups. In this case the goal is often to expand the range of discussion by bringing in new questions rather than to ensure a focus on predetermined questions. A similar principle applies across a set of exploratory groups, as the insights learned in one group may lead to new questions in future groups, while questions that have been exhausted in prior groups may be dropped in favor of new lines of exploration. Because of this variation from group to group, the analysis of exploratory groups is understandably less straightforward than in more structured forms of focus groups. If the research goals include a thorough analysis of the spectrum of ideas and perspectives revealed in the discussions, then an exploratory design should be matched to a relatively lengthy time slot for analysis.

Finally there is the loosely structured approach, which gives every sign of producing unfocused focus groups. That would undoubtedly occur if this approach were taken without regard to the match between the topic and the participants' ability to discuss it. In many cases leaving both the topic and its management largely up to the participants would produce halting, meandering discussions that would be of little use for any coherent research goal. Consequently, loosely structured groups are most appropriate when the participants have a strong concern for the topic at hand. When the group has sufficient experience with and interest in the subject of the research, then it is feasible to let them undertake a self-managed exploration of the topic. Like the phenomenological approach, this exploration will let them recount their own experiences in their own words; like the exploratory approach, it will let them consider a broad sweep of topics.

Loosely structured groups still require considerable forethought on the part of the researcher. As with phenomenological groups, a moderator should give the groups instructions on self-management and should be on hand during the discussion. A particularly useful tactic is to validate the expression of differences within the group, using instructions such as, "We want to hear about as many different experiences as we possibly can. So if you are listening to someone and thinking, 'That wasn't how it was for me,' then that's exactly when we need you to speak up and tell us about your feelings and experiences."

The fact that four distinctly different types of focus groups can be generated using only a consideration of the structure dimension demonstrates the range of designs that are possible. The choice among these four types cannot, however, be made in a vacuum. Although the presentation of the structure dimension has proceeded as if this decision could be made independently, the reality is that many design decisions are interdependent. This interdependency will be emphasized throughout the remainder of the chapter.

## How Large Should Each Group Be?

After group structure, group size is probably the next most important design decision. Unquestionably, the minimum size for a group interview is at least two participants; oddly enough, however, little consideration has been given to very small "groups" within the focus group literature. As a practical minimum most treatments of focus groups assume at least four participants. Although it is evident that a lively group discussion can emerge among four people, it remains unclear whether groups with either two or three participants are focus groups or something else.

The high end of the size range is even murkier. Certainly groups with a dozen participants have different dynamics than groups of four or five, but this provides little guidance on what the theoretical maximum size is. To see that some form of group interview is possible with very large groups, it is sufficient to note that many of the practitioners of focus group research are university professors who routinely attempt to foster discussions in classes with far more than 10 or 12 students. Still, for most purposes the practical range of focus groups size is from around 4 to around 15, with the rule of thumb pointing to a somewhat narrower portion of this range.

The key difference between large and small groups is in the dynamics of their discussions. Smaller groups tend to generate more intense and detailed discussions, with more information available about the point of view of each separate participant. Consequently, when the research calls for delving more deeply into the detailed experiences and feelings of individuals, smaller groups are preferred. Larger groups are more likely to produce a steady flow of brief, loosely connected remarks, with some members contributing rather little to the group. When the research calls for generating a number of different ideas and possibilities, then larger groups are preferred.

As with group structure, the fact that group size affects the basic nature of the data to be collected means that it has implications for many other aspects of the research design. First among these is the connection between group size and group structure. Unfortunately no succinct answer exists to the obvious question of whether more structure is necessary in small groups or in large groups. Instead size and structure are intersecting dimensions, and it is possible to run a more structured or less structured group at any point in the size continuum. For smaller groups more structure is likely to be necessary when the participants do not have a lot of experience with or interest in the topic. With such low-intensity topics, small groups are particularly vulnerable to problems in group dynamics, and a moderator may be necessary either to encourage discussion or to keep one or two individuals from dominating. With larger groups the issue of structure is more likely to be one of keeping order in the group, especially when the participants are interested in the topic. With a high-intensity topic, large groups may break into several separate conversations if no structure is imposed through either predetermined questions or external management of the group interaction.

Group size also raises issues that cut across the other design dimensions. With regard to group composition, it is less difficult to run a homogeneous group than a heterogeneous one at any point on the size continuum. If one is dealing with heterogeneous groups, it is usually easier to rely on the loose, less involved discussion of larger groups rather than confront the problems with group dynamics in smaller mixed groups. A similar principle applies to strangers and friends: Strangers will present more difficulty in small groups, due to the problem of generating a discussion; friends will present more difficulty in large groups, due to the problem of maintaining an orderly group discussion rather than a general buzz of multiple conversations. Finally the size of groups may or may not be connected closely to the number of groups, depending on the availability of participants. When an unlimited number of participants is available, then one is free to make group size decisions on other bases. If only a limited number of participants is available, however, one must consider the difference between running a few large groups versus many small groups even though the total number of participants might be identical.

## How Should the Group Be Composed?

It is important not to confuse issues of group composition with sampling issues, such as who the participants should be and how they should be located. Instead the question here is how the membership in the focus groups should be constructed for a given sample. The rules of thumb call for maintaining two basic aspects of group composition: The members of the groups should be relatively homogeneous, and they should be unacquainted with each other.

With regard to homogeneity, the rule of thumb against mixing differing types of participants arises from the fact that people are most likely to feel comfortable in discussions with others whom they perceive to be similar to themselves. In other words, homogeneous groups are more likely to generate an easily flowing discussion on a topic of shared interest. When the goal is to achieve smooth, conversationlike group dynamics, then a homogeneous group is the appropriate design decision. Mixed groups do have potential advantages, however. In particular the obvious existence of differences within a group often encourages participants to express a wider range of feelings and experiences. In addition, encountering different points of view typically leads participants to explore why they think as they do. When the goal is a broader range of ideas or a deeper reflection on the bases for beliefs, then heterogeneous groups offer a distinct advantage.

Of course groups are always "mixed" with regard to something, so the issue is which aspects of group composition must be controlled. In making this decision, it is useful to distinguish between comparative designs and those that involve different population segments. The discussion in the previous paragraph is most likely to apply to a segmented population, where different subgroups divide the sample by sex, age, race, social class, and so on. In such a case the goal is to mix or match participants to generate the most productive group dynamics. In comparative research the need to maintain homogeneity within groups is often a basic part of the design. In such a case the goal is to get the purest expression of the point of view of each type of participant.

Turning to the question of whether to use strangers or acquaintances, the rule of thumb points to the fact that using participants who do not know each other eliminates many potential problems. For one thing, friendship groups have informal norms that limit and direct what is said, thus leaving implicit many of the things a researcher might wish to observe. For another, it is typically easier to manage the group dynamics among strangers, since groups composed of friends have a tendency to break into private conversations.

In reality, whether strangers are used often depends on the practicalities of sample availability rather than on abstract issues of research design. The distorted dynamics of groups that include acquaintances may be a small price to pay for ready access to a rare sample. Other design considerations may also override the preference for strangers. In particular, when the preference is strong for running self-managed groups, this is often easier to accomplish when the group members are already acquainted. It is also worth noting that some research questions may call for studying group processes that depend on preexisting friendships. Thus informal norms in friendship groups are not a problem if the operation of these norms is precisely what the research is designed to study; for example, as in examining the role of peer groups in behavior changes such as smoking cessation.

## How Many Groups Should There Be?

The number of groups used in a project depends on how clear the research goals are and how diverse the population is. If the understanding of the results that the research is to produce is well developed, and if the population is not divided into too many segments or geographical sites, then it is usually safe to rely on the rule of thumb that four to six groups are sufficient. One common temptation is to run a few groups, see how the results are turning out, and then add more groups as necessary. The problem with this strategy is that it can get out of control; Feig (1989) reports the case of a marketing project that ended up running over 60 groups in this fashion. Pursuing an open-ended number of groups is a workable strategy only if one in fact has criteria for assessing "how the results are turning out." Most researchers have no problem avoiding this strategy once they realize the additional time and money involved in not only collecting but also analyzing an unnecessarily large number of groups.

In designing a research project with fewer than the typical number of groups, the practical minimum that one should consider is two. Research using only one group is highly vulnerable because the researcher has no way of knowing the extent to which the data from that group reflect something about the unique mix of personalities and circumstances that went into it. If the same content emerges quite clearly in two different groups, then the researcher is on more solid ground in concluding that the desired data have been captured. The most acceptable justification for running a single group is a rare or inaccessible study population; in that case the single group represents the best available data, and it is better to have half a loaf than none at all.

Exploratory research is likely to require more groups than the norm because of the benefits from using less structured approaches in this case. Allowing the questions to evolve from group to group and permitting the group to seek its own direction in the discussions aid the exploration of a topic but only at the cost of relatively inefficient groups. Gaining a sense of stability about the findings uncovered in unstructured groups is likely to require a larger number of observations. In other words a highly structured group is likely to be more productive than its less structured equivalent, so any project, exploratory or otherwise, that uses less structured groups will often require more groups than are indicated by the rule of thumb.

Two other cases that require a larger number of groups are (a) investigating several topics simultaneously and (b) comparing several subgroups. For multiple topics the wide-ranging discussions that are necessary will yield correspondingly less discussion about any single topic in each group. Thus more groups are necessary to ensure an adequate volume of material on each topic. For multiple sample segments, one has to gather enough material from each segment to compare it with the others. When comparing different groups, it is a virtual necessity to have at least two groups of each type, due once again to the uncertainties associated with the data from a single group. For this and many other purposes, it is important to remember that it is the group rather than the participant that is the unit of analysis in focus group research. Hence the original rule of thumb can be expanded to suggest that comparative designs require four to six groups in each sample segment.

In concluding this look at the four basic design dimensions, it is necessary to say something about how the design dimensions intersect. Although the discussion of each dimension has included a consideration of how it relates to the others, this is still an oversimplification. The reality is that all of the dimensions have to be considered simultaneously for any particular project. Such interdependencies in research design are likely to be the rule rather than the exception in all fields, and focus groups are no exception. At this point rather little can be said about research design for focus groups at this level of complexity, so it is appropriate to end this summary of design issues by noting that we still have much to accomplish.

## Discussion and Conclusions

Up to this point the discussion has followed the traditional stipulation that research designs must flow from research questions. While the priority of the research question can never be disregarded, a number of other factors influence the kind of project one is capable of executing. At a minimum the amount of money and the time available are powerful constraints on research design.

When finances limit the design of focus groups, it is often necessary to absorb some of the personnel expenses. Professionals typically charge several hundred dollars per group to do the moderating and analysis. This is the largest expense in focus groups, so the greatest saving is to have members of the research team perform these functions. Although moderating is a highly specialized skill, it is not uncommon to find team members who have experience working with groups. Such semiskilled moderators are most appropriate when the groups have less structure with regard to group dynamics, so groups in this format can cut costs. The trade-off with unstructured groups is that they are more difficult to analyze, so little is saved unless the analysis is also done in-house. In fact most social scientists are likely to do their own analyses, especially if they have experience with analyzing other forms of qualitative data. If this is the case, it also creates a halfway option: paying a professional moderator a lesser amount to conduct the groups but not to do the analysis.

Conducting the groups and analyzing the data are the time-consuming aspects of focus group research. To cut time on the former, it may be possible to assemble a large number of participants at a single site and to run several groups simultaneously. Such a strategy often involves using a preexisting group, which also minimizes the time spent on recruitment. To save time in analysis, it is necessary to eliminate the detailed coding of transcripts. One option is to have members of the research team attend the groups, make notes, and then meet in groups of their own to discuss their observations. Another option is to do the analysis by listening to tapes. This option eliminates the time (and expense) involved in transcription, but listening to tapes is much slower and less efficient than reading transcripts. In large cities a better time-saving alternative is to contract with a professional typing service for rapid production of the transcriptions. If one is using transcripts, running more structured groups will save time, as this practice generates orderly transcripts that are more easily compared across groups.

Designing research to save either time or money essentially imposes constraints on the choices one can make, but the central issue is still making choices. This emphasis on making choices, like the emphasis on using the research question as a basis for design decisions, has placed another limitation on this presentation. Discussing every design issue in terms of a decision among alternatives gives a sense that any given project has to be done one way or the other. Actually focus group designs are considerably more flexible than that.

One way to take advantage of this flexibility is through projects that combine several different designs, such as structured and unstructured groups, in a single study. For example, one could begin with a first set of two or three very unstructured groups to determine what the appropriate questions are for subsequent groups; then a second set of groups could be run that was structured with regard to the questions but still relatively unstructured with regard to group dynamics; and a final set of groups could be run in a highly structured fashion in order to pursue any issues of further interest to the researchers. Another design dimension in which a combination of different types of groups can be useful is the homogeneity of the group composition. Where issues of homogeneity and heterogeneity are of particular interest, one can compare sets of mixed and unmixed groups.

This emphasis on flexibility is an appropriate conclusion for this chapter. Focus groups are still an evolving method, and it is crucial that this development be encouraged. The movement away from unquestioned rules of thumb toward conscious decisions among alternatives is one way to create a broader range of focus group designs. This strategy does, however, carry the danger of simply introducing a new orthodoxy. It would be a serious mistake if the discussion here was misinterpreted as constituting a new set of standards for focus group research, rather than out the gamut of choices associated with this technique.

What should the future produce in terms of research design with focus groups? The promotion of consistent and coherent guidelines for assessing design decisions is certainly one desirable goal. But we cannot allow this striving toward consistency to stifle creativity. In my ideal view, a reading of this chapter 10 years hence should reveal two kinds of progress. First, the experientially based guidelines summarized here will have been replaced with solid results from methodological research. Second, the range of design alternatives considered here will have been greatly expanded by the inventiveness of a new generation of researchers. This is an ambitious agenda, but one that clearly highlights the opportunities for those of us who wish to design research using focus groups.

# References

Basch, C. E. (1987). Focus group interview: An underutilized research technique for improving theory and practice in health education. *Health Education Quarterly, 14,* 411-448.

Calder, B. J. (1977). Focus groups and the nature of qualitative marketing research. *Journal of Marketing Research, 14,* 353-364.

Feig, B. (1989). How to run a focus group: Focus groups become hocus-pocus when researchers manipulate them to make a client look good. *American Demographics, 11,* 36-37.

Fern, E. F. (1982). The use of focus groups for idea generation: The effects of group size, acquaintanceship, and moderator on response quantity and quality. *Journal of Marketing Research, 19,* 1-13.

Flaskerud J. H., & Rush, C. E. (1989). AIDS and traditional health beliefs and practices of black women. *Nursing Research, 38,* 210-215.

Frey, J. H., & Fontana, A. (1991). The group interview in social research. *Social Science Journal, 28,* 175-187.

Goldman A. E., & McDonald, S. S. (1987). *The group depth interview.* Englewood Cliffs, NJ: Prentice Hall.

Greenbaum, I. L. (1987). *The practical handbook and guide to focus group research.* Lexington, MA: Lexington.

Howland J., Sargent, J., Weitzman, M., Mangione, T., Ebert, R., Mauceri, M., & Bond, M. (1989). Barriers to bicycle helmet use among children. *American Journal of Diseases of Children, 143,* 741-744.

Joseph, J. G., Emmons, C. A., Kessler, R. C., Wortman, C. B., O'Brien, K., Hocker, W. T., & Schaefer, C. (1984). Coping with the threat of AIDS: An approach to psychosocial assessment. *American Psychologist, 39,* 1297-1302.

Krueger, R. A. (1988). *Focus groups: A practical guide for applied research.* Newbury Park, CA: Sage.

Morgan, D. L. (1988). *Focus groups as qualitative research.* (Sage University Paper Series on Qualitiative Research Methods, Vol. 16). Newbury Park, CA: Sage.

Morgan, D. L. (1989a). Adjustment to widowhood: Do social networks really help? *The Gerontologist, 29,* 101-107.

Morgan, D. L. (1989b). *Caregivers for elderly Alzheimer's victims: A comparison of caregiving in the home and in institutions.* Final Report to the AARP/Andrus Foundation.

Morgan, D. L. (1990). Combining the strengths of social networks, social support, and personal relationships. In S. Duck (Ed.), *Personal relationships and social support.* Newbury Park, CA: Sage.

Morgan, D. L., & Spanish, M. T. (1985). Social interaction and the cognitive organization of health-relevant behavior. *Sociology of Health and Illness, 7,* 401-422.

Taylor, T. R. (1989). Pity the poor gatekeeper: A transatlantic perspective on cost containment in clinical practice. *British Medical Journal, 299,* 1323-1325.

# 16 Depth Interviewing: The Long Interview Approach

WILLIAM L. MILLER
BENJAMIN F. CRABTREE

## Introduction

Listening, along with seeing and touching, is one of the primary sources of information about the world. As a data collection tool, the interview represents an attempt to "standardize" listening in the interest of scientific knowing. This chapter details the Long Interview as an example of a semistructured in-depth interview approach to collecting data in primary care research and illustrates the approach using a pain research project.

In the context of primary care research, how do doctors and patients think about pain? Our present knowledge about pain informs us that seeing (e.g., through observation or pain-drawings) and touching (e.g., through examination or experimental stimulation) are inadequate sources of data (Fields, 1987; Frank, Moll, & Hurt, 1982). Pain is a physiosubjective experience, and understanding it requires asking both patients and physicians about their experiences of pain. Thus, how are we to listen? We can position ourselves within social situations in which people are in pain and eavesdrop on the conversations that spontaneously arise, or we can enter casually into these same conversations. When pain is mentioned within the discourse, we can even interrupt and informally explore the topic further. These unstructured approaches are informative, and we encourage social scientists to pursue them. For the primary care researcher, however, they are usually too time-consuming. The most often used alternative approach (described more fully in Chapter 10) is to formally develop a common set of questions, lists, or ratings about pain and to expose selected respondents to these same sets of stimuli (Frank et al., 1982). This structured approach, however, runs the high risk of putting the researcher's own concerns into the mouths of the respondents and never learning the latter's own perception and understanding about pain.

Fortunately primary care researchers with limited resources can also opt for a semistructured, depth interview approach. This method combines the practical advantages of the structured approach with the open-ended discourse style of unstructured listening. We used the Long Interview, a specific depth interview technique, to listen to six family physician-patient pairs from a small suburban community in north central Connecticut. The goal was to identify and compare their understandings and experiences of pain. The depth interview is a powerful data collection tool when the focus of inquiry is narrow, the respondents represent a homogeneous group and are familiar and comfortable with the interview as a means of communication, and the goal is to generate dominant themes and narratives.

In the remainder of this chapter we will demonstrate the "doing" of this Long Interview, illustrating each step with the pain research outlined above. In order to provide context, we will first briefly review the types of strategies for interviewing and then contrast the interview with other kinds of communication.

## Interviewing Strategies

Interviewing strategies are commonly organized on the basis of structure. Table 16.1 presents types of interviews within the context of other data collection tools. The table distinguishes informal everyday talk occurring in participant observation fieldwork, unstructured interviews focusing on a particular topic, semistructured interviews using interview guides, and structured interviews utilizing interview schedules that standardize the questions or stimuli and maximize interviewer control. Informal and unstructured interviews, such as those taking place in situational conversations or planned unstructured encounters, possess high contextual validity, especially when linked with other data collection tools (Kirk & Miller, 1986). Their reliability, however, is poor. Structured interviews, which include surveys, free listing, pile sorts, and rank order methods (Weller & Romney, 1988) are much more reliable but frequently possess dubious validity unless carefully developed from more unstructured fieldwork methods. Semistructured interviews include life histories (Denzin, 1989b; Watson & Watson-Franke, 1985), key informant interviews (Ellen, 1984), depth or focused interviews (Douglas, 1985;

**Table 16.1** Data Collection Tools for Primary Care Research

UNOBTRUSIVE
   Direct (Reactive)
OBSERVATION
   Unstructured
   Structured (e.g., Mapping, Category systems, Checklists, Rating scales, Kinesics, Proxemics)
   Participant
RECORDINGS
   (e.g., Audio, Visual, A/V)
DIARIES
INTERVIEWING
   Informal (e.g., Eavesdropping, Everyday conversation)
   Unstructured
   Semistructured (Interview guide)
      Key informant/Elite
      Depth/Focused (e.g., Long Interview, Focus Groups)
      Life History (Biography)
      Ethnoscience ("Ethnographic")
      Critical incidents technique
      Projective techniques
      Other (e.g., Ecomap, Life space, Genogram, Kingram)
   Sturctured (Interview Schedule)
      Free listing
      Pile sorts/Triad Comparisons (Q sorts)
      Rank order methods (e.g., Paired comparisions, Balanced incomplete block design)
      Surveys (e.g., Open-ended, Factorial, Forced choice)
QUESTIONNAIRES
   Surveys(e.g., Ratings, Likert, Semantic differential, Cumulative/Guttman)
   Tests (e.g., Dichotomous format, Multiple choice, Fill-in-the-blank,
      Matchings, Estimation/Magnitude, Pick N, Sentence ccompletion)
ARCHIVES/DOCUMENTS
CULTURAL PRODUCTS
   (e.g., Physical artifacts, Music/Art/Dance, Film/Fiction/folktales/Games/Jokes)
BIOPHYSICAL MEASURES

Merton, Fiske, & Kendall, 1956), critical incident techniques (Dunn & Hamilton, 1986), ethnoscientific approaches (Spradley, 1979), projective techniques (Pelto & Pelto, 1978), and other techniques specifically developed for primary care such as the genogram (McGoldrick & Gerson, 1985) and life space (Blake & Bertuso, 1988). All of these approaches are most trustworthy when used for exploratory studies or for discovering the perceptions of specific individuals.

## The Interview as a
## Communication Event

The traditional understanding of the interview assumes it is primarily a behaviorial event consisting of informational verbal exchange. The interviewer supplies a stimulus and the interviewee responds; each question and answer is assumed to be independently meaningful and isolatable and can be coded and counted accordingly. It is becoming increasingly clear that all of these assumptions are false. In every interview there also are nonverbal interchanges and a continuous exchange of multilayered messages being differentially perceived (Mishler, 1986). The questions and transmissions are complex, ambiguous, and jointly constructed from the context of the discourse. Both the interviewer and the respondent have multiple social roles beyond their roles in this situation, and these different roles influence the many different motivations each has for engaging in the interview. Some of these interactional goals include requests, expression, politeness, persuasion, attention, exerting authority, therapy, ritual, evaluation, and/or reference to specific knowledge. The interviewer's goal is knowledge, but this goal may not be shared by the respondent.

The research interview is a special type of communication event; it is not political oratory, storytelling, a lecture, a small group seminar, or a clinical encounter. Interview discourse occurs within a specific social situation consisting of a physical place, activities, and participants who have their own social role identities and interactional goals. A second context for any communication event is the communication or discourse itself. This includes the form of the message (verbal, gestural, etc.); the actual message or sign; and the person, object, event, or process represented by the sign (Briggs, 1986; Gottlieb, 1986).

The research interview as a communication event presumes hierarchical interviewer-respondent role relations. Rules exist for introducing new topics, taking turns, and judging the relevance of statements. Expectations also exist for etiquette, linguistic forms, and an understanding that the major purpose of the interaction is to provide referential information. When communicating in "the interview," the respondent talks the most; turn order is fixed; the length of exchange is specified; topics are fixed; and turn allocation and interview rapport are controlled by the interviewer (Sacks, Schegloff, & Jefferson, 1974). This is quite different from everyday conversation.

A profound implication of understanding the interview as a communication event is the clarification of when and which type of interview to use as a data collection tool. *The interview becomes an appropriate tool only if interviewing is a known communication routine of the respondent and if it is a culturally appropriate communication form for the topic of interest* (Briggs, 1986). As Briggs notes, learning how to ask requires that we first identify the different ways in which people communicate, and then decide on the appropriate research methods.

In the remainder of this chapter we will concentrate only on one particular type of depth interview, the Long Interview as presented by McCracken (1988). The Long Interview primarily focuses on a narrow, specific topic within a larger context and uses open, direct, verbal questions, which elicit stories and case narratives. We chose this data collection tool in our pain study because (a) we knew our potential respondents are familiar and comfortable with the interview as a communication event; (b) discourse about pain in the study community often takes the form of stories (by patients) and of cases (by physicians); (c) the discourse about pain between doctors and patients usually occurs within an interview format using direct, verbal questions; (d) our study was exploratory; and (e) our goal was to discover individuals' perceptions and narrative understandings about pain.

## The Long Interview

The complete interview-to-transcription process involves a series of carefully designed steps. Briefly, an interview guide is constructed following an extensive literature review and a systematic uncovering of the preconceptions of the members of the research team. Once the guide is complete, a pilot interview is performed, a purposive sample of approximately 6 to 10 subjects is identified, and informed consent is obtained. Interviews are audiotaped and later transcribed. The analysis of these transcripts is discussed in Chapter 17.

### LITERATURE REVIEW: THE DISCOVERY OF ANALYTIC CATEGORIES

McCracken (1988) intends that the literature review would identify the existing descriptive, theoretical, and analytic categories for the research topic. The review needs to be broad. The initial goal is to search out the literature's assumptions and expectations and then to identify key conceptual domains around which an interview guide can be developed. The final goal of the entire research enterprise is to generalize the specific research findings back to this theoretical literature. In our review of the literature on pain, we discovered that most of the articles and other written material are broadly categorized into the domains of "socialization," "pain types," "types of pain people," and "management of pain" (Barnhouse, Kilodychuk, Pankratz, & Olinger, 1988; Diamond & Grauer, 1986; Fagerhaugh & Strauss, 1977; Hilbert, 1984; Kleinman & Good, 1985; Kotarba & Seidel, 1984; Perry, 1985).

## UNCOVERING PRECONCEPTIONS:
## THE DISCOVERY
## OF CULTURAL CATEGORIES

Cultural categories refer to the professional and everyday or "common sense" understandings that both the researchers and the respondents have about the research topic and methods. In order to "bring out" the researcher's preconceptions, members of the research team must be willing to expose their inner thoughts and emotions both to themselves and to the other members of the team. In our study each person inventoried her or his own past pain incidents, associations, and assumptions. This process is usually very painful and discomforting, especially when hidden personal feelings and value inconsistencies are uncovered. This cultural self-exploration is important later for text analysis when the revealed cultural categories influence interpretation of the collected data. The self-exploration also prepares a reservoir of empathy for the researcher when the respondent shares similar thoughts and emotions.

McCracken (1988) focuses on the research team as the sole source for these discovered cultural categories. We recommend that the discovery of cultural categories be expanded to include (a) a review of the ethnographic reports on the culture or subculture of the respondents, and (b) preliminary direct contact with individuals from the cultural group being studied. One approach to discovering the cultural categories of the respondents is to convene a focus group (see Chapter 15). Finally it is important to investigate any sociolinguistic studies of the respondents' cultural group to make sure the interview is an appropriate tool for investigating the research topic, particularly if this group is not well acculturated into Western society. The cultural self-exploration of our own pain experiences and understandings substantiated the domains discovered in the literature review.

## THE DRAMATIC OUTLINE:
## CONSTRUCTING AN INTERVIEW GUIDE

The Long Interview is organized around an interview guide consisting of relatively closed introductory questions and a few (three to six) open-ended "grand tour" questions followed by more specific prompts or probes. The stage is set by rapport-building biographical questions, followed by the introduction of research themes through questions designed to elicit narratives that detail the informant's conception of the identified domains.

The first set of questions in the Long Interview is composed of standard biographical ones, which ask for short, structured, direct answers. These introductory questions serve the following six functions: (a) establish interview style, (b) build rapport, (c) jog the respondent's memory, (d) build a bridge to intimacy, (e) provide context data for analysis, and (f) weave a discourse context for the topical research questions. These 10-20 minutes spent talking about birthplace, family, religion, and occupation create a climate of trust, communication, and self-disclosure. The interviewing couple is prepared for the grand tour.

Grand tour questions are direct, easy to answer, nonthreatening, open, and descriptive and seek to elicit key terms and major features or attributes about people, acts, time, goals, and feelings (Spradley, 1979). A good grand tour question gets the respondent into the topic of interest and gets the interviewer out of the way. In order to succeed, the question must be broad, use clearly defined terms, provide necessary time and space perspectives, supply needed facts, stimulate memory, avoid jargon and emotionally loaded words, be easily and clearly understandable, delimit the scope of the question, avoid suggesting an answer, and arouse the respondent's interest and motivation (Gordon, 1975). The grand tour questions are based on the categories discovered during the literature reviews and cultural category explorations. They are designed to provide answers that are ultimately generalizable to the theoretical literature and yet are the respondent's own.

In our pain study, the four broad categories found in the literature review were consistent with those discovered in the search for cultural categories. Thus four grand tour questions were developed for the interview guide based on these domains. The final wording of each question followed lengthy group discussions. For example, the initial wording of the pain management question was, "Would you explain your management approach to pain?" Group analysis revealed that this question presumes respondents have already described *what* they do and are now to explain *why* they do it, when we really wanted a description of the former. The word *management* represents confusing jargon from medical, political, and economic perspectives. The question is also not clear about whose pain is to be managed and for whom the description is intended—the interviewer or some other audience. In response to these issues the final question form became, "Would you *describe for me how you decide what to do* when *you* have pain?" The italics identify the specific changes.

Once launched on the grand tour, the interviewer must be prepared to keep the story flowing without influencing the content. This is accomplished through the use of floating prompts. Seven such prompts include *silence*, or the permissive pause, which gives control to the respondent, enhances spontaneity, and creates a thoughtful mood; the *attentive lean*, in which the interviewer leans toward the respondent with an affirmative head nod; the *eyebrow flash*; an *affirmative noise*, such as "uhhuh"; the *echo prompt*, or repeating the last word spoken by the respondent in an interrogative style; the *reflective summary*, in which the interviewer summarizes the respondent's last statement; and *recapitulation*, or representing in summary form something mentioned earlier in the interview (Bernard, 1988; Gordon, 1975; Schatzman & Strauss, 1973; Whyte, 1984).

A successful grand tour facilitated by strategically placed floating prompts elicits key terms and features, but not all of these terms will be fully detailed. Details are obtained through the use of planned probes. The most commonly used planned probes are *category questions*, which simply seek elaboration and/or clarification of all the parts, settings, relationships, activities, and the relative worth or value of the domain being discussed; these include the what else, where, when, how, why, and why important questions. Another common planned probe is the *contrast question*, which seeks to clarify the similarities and differences between two key terms or features: "What is the difference between [blank] and [blank]?" (Spradley, 1979). Additional probes can include the *hypothetical question, devil's advocate questions, special incident probes, posing the ideal probes,* and *phased assertion*, or baiting, which should be used only as a last resort (Bernard, 1988; Schatzman & Strauss, 1973). Probes must be as carefully worded as the grand tour questions and must avoid leading the respondent (e.g., see Example #1).

### Example #1

I:   (Interviewer) Well, see if you can tell me. . . Think of something that's. . . And you can tell me as a story. I want you to start at the beginning and tell me a tale, like, "I woke up in pain," and so on, or whatever the situation is.

R:  (Respondent) Well, back then, then I'd be limited because there is nothing to tell there. I wake up and it's there. (Story continues. . .)

In this segment of the transcript, the interviewer is trying to get the respondent to recite a narrative about her experiences with pain. Unfortunately, however, the respondent may have chosen this "wake up" story because the interviewer suggested it.

The final step in constructing an interview guide is to conduct one or more pilot interviews, usually with friends. This process will help in finalizing the sequence and wording of the grand tour questions and will suggest additional planned probes. It also serves as a training tool for the interviewers.

## SELECTING THE ACTORS: SAMPLING

For semistructured depth interviews, the selection of respondents should maximize the richness of information pertinent to the research question. As such the sampling strategy should be purposeful and not random. Patton (1987) discusses several types of information-rich sampling strategies, including extreme or deviant case, maximum variation, homogeneous, typical case, critical case, snowball or chain, criterion, confirmatory or disconfirming case, sampling politically important cases, and convenience sampling. One or more of these can be used, depending on the particular research situation; however, note that convenience sampling is the least desirable and should generally be avoided.

In our research on pain, we used a combination of homogeneous, criterion, and snowball sampling. We wanted individuals from a homogenous community, who had had recent exposure to pain, and their family physicians. Therefore we selected the first six family physicians from a small homogeneous community and asked them each to provide the name of a patient over age 21 who had been discharged from a hospital within the previous 2 weeks. The result is our six family physician-patient pairs.

## STAGING THE SCENE:
## THE INTERVIEW SETTING

Once the dramatic outline is complete and the actors selected, the interview scene must be staged or set. The interview is a staged communication event—a purposefully situated process (Douglas, 1985). Each social situation or scene has its own culturally prescribed norms of nonverbal and verbal interactions that influence the interpretation of what is expressed (Briggs, 1986). Since the goal of semistructured depth interviews involves maximizing the flow of accurate respondent-derived information, most such interviews should occur in a "grass hut" setting—that is, the usual, everyday location where the research topic is discussed, as opposed to a "white room" or sterile context site. Good lighting (to facilitate observation on nonverbal communication), a minimum of external disturbance (sound or activity), privacy, a face-to-face encounter with a 6 to 8-foot separation, and well-mannered informality are also helpful staging parameters (Douglas, 1985).

For our pain study, we elected to interview the family physicians at their offices, where they routinely engage in private interviews with their patients about pain. Interviews with patients took place in the privacy of their homes.

The preinterview contact has six goals: (a) introduce yourself; that is, identify role and give name, (b) identify sponsorship, (c) explain purpose, (d) explain selection of respondent, (e) assure anonymity, and (f) obtain informed consent. The interviewer may also wish to discuss note taking, recording, and anticipated length of interview (Gordon, 1975). It is usually better to do all this at least a day before the actual interview, as this prevents any possible ego threat at the time of the interview. The preinterview contact also involves a negotiation-type of discourse, which is quite different from the interview discourse. In our pain study, this preinterview contact took place by telephone usually a week before the interview. Remember to bring extra batteries for the tape recorder.

### LET THE PLAY BEGIN:
### THE INTERVIEW PROCESS

As we have presented it, the semistructured depth interview is a constructed dialogue focused on a creative search for mutual personal understanding of a research topic. It requires sincerity, cooperative mutual disclosure, and warmth (Douglas, 1985). The discourse must be open; no two interviews will be the same. Thus the interviewer needs to be open to the pain and uncertainty of self-discovery. The interviewer, not the research guide, is the research instrument. The interviewer's role is to assume a low-profile stance to put the informant at ease, to acknowledge the value of the information, to empathize with the respondent, and to reinforce the continuance of the conversation.

The interview is as paradoxical a tool as the human existence it seeks to probe. Having just pleaded for the interviewer to engage the respondent with warmth and intimacy, we now argue for the interviewer to manufacture and maintain distance within this relationship (McCracken, 1988). Phenomenologists refer to this distancing as "bracketing"—putting the self aside so that a phenomenon can be experienced as it is (Denzin, 1989a). This process requires the self-understanding undertaken earlier when discovering cultural categories. The interview is a dance of intimacy and distancing, which creates a dramatic space where the respondent discloses his or her inner thoughts and feelings and the interviewer knowingly hears and facilitates the story and recognizes and repairs any communication missteps. Humor, gentle surprise, and the use of metaphors (such as our dramaturgical one) are a few helpful techniques for manufacturing distance (McCracken, 1988). See Example #2.

*Example #2*

R: I think losing a child must be, must be terrible, really terrible. I think a husband and wife always expect, some day you're going to lose each other. I would hope if I had to lose one of those four kids, I could handle that. They're nice kids, they really are. I sound like a mother! (Laughs.)

I: (Laughs.) What are mothers for? Let's talk a little bit. . . You were telling me about the pain if you lost a child or pain for a death. Could you tell me, from your experience, what the usual or typical kinds of pain are?

A good interview has a slow, progressive flow and should maximize the facilitators and minimize the inhibitors of this flow. Gordon (1975) describes four inhibitors that limit the willingness or motivation of the informant to provide information: (a) competing demands for time, (b) ego threats (evasion, denial, minimization, confession, and depersonalization), (c) etiquette, and (d) recollection of a traumatic event. He also mentions four inhibitors that limit the ability of the informant to provide information: (a) forgetting, (b) chronological confusion, (c) inferential confusion, and (d) unconscious behavior. Facilitators discussed by Gordon to maximize the interview flow include: (a) fulfilling expectations, (b) recognition, (c) altruistic appeals, (d) sympathetic understanding, (e) new experience, (f) catharsis, (g) need for meaning, and (h) extrinsic rewards.

Judicious use of prompts and probes as the grand tour responses evolve is essential for maintaining the progressive flow of conversation. Two general rules of thumb are (a) avoid dominance-submission or parent-child games (Douglas, 1985), and (b) use the least direct probe necessary. Begin with silence and slowly progress to self-disclosure. Paddling in the flow of interview discourse is much like paddling a canoe: In slow, smooth water, paddle harder with more directness; when in choppy water, just use the paddle gently to maintain course (Whyte, 1984).

Not all interviews proceed smoothly, and the interviewer should have several strategies for dealing with the different types of resistance that occasionally emerge. If a fearful respondent wants to know why you are taking notes, just say why. For the commonly encountered "I don't remember," a permissive pause often brings results. If a respondent becomes tongue-tied, use a reflective probe (immediate elaboration). Steering runaways back on course often necessitates a gentle change of topic. Gordon (1975) suggests that when a reluctant respondent says "I don't know anything," the interviewer can use retrospective elaboration and encouragement. In Example #3 the respondent is having difficulty with a question eliciting information about what doctors should think about when dealing with pain.

*Example #3*

R: With a doctor relieving my pain?

I: Whatever occurs to you.

R: Um. Maybe I'm not getting the question right.

I: Could be. Let's start with. . .

R: You mean if a doctor thought the patient might become addicted to a pain medicine, he might not give it to them? He'd have to know his patients pretty well. Still, I suppose he'd still have to give you something to relieve whatever you had. I don't know what to tell you on that one.

I: If you went to a doctor with pain, what would you hope that the doctor would do for you?

R: Well, I would hope that if I went to him with pain, that he would give me something that would relieve it. And if it was something that was going to continue, that he'd tell me what he was going to do about it like an operation or something like that. I'd want it right away. I wouldn't want to stay on medication.

Here an encouraging reframing keeps the discourse flowing.

The alert interviewer is also continuously evaluating the content of the ongoing discourse: listening for key terms, watching for changes in the type of communication, such as switching from interview discourse to performative discourse, and listening for possible misunderstandings. It is also important to identify those times when the respondent is attempting to create an impression or self-presentation image. All people have aspects of themselves that remain outside of self-awareness— what Douglas (1985) calls our personal "black holes." Sensitive interviewers can recognize a respondent's (and their own) black holes when they encounter persistent topic avoidance, exaggerated behavior or responses, or an inappropriate lack of emotional display. These are signals to ease up and to go more slowly, to manufacture distance, and possibly to use self-disclosure (e.g., see Example #4).

*Example #4*

R: Well I think (laughs) you've brought back a few memories I'd forgotten I even had! The first time I ever had real pain was when I had the first baby. And Joseph was very. . . He was the second one. Sue was a tough one. She was the last one. She couldn't make up her mind if she wanted to come out or not. (Laughs.) Like I say, I've never really thought about pain until this week when you called and asked me if I would talk to you and I thought, what can I tell her about pain? I don't even have headaches. So I guess there's a lot to be said about it.

I: What's it like to think about it?

R: I don't know because I never think about it.

I: Now that you are thinking about it. (Laughs.)

R: Yes, right. Um, I think even as much compassion as I have for Charlie, for all this length of time, I would even have a little more for him, because I know he doesn't have any pain with the ah, you know, the stoma and all that sort of thing. But I often think when I change it for him, if there's pain there he's not telling me about it. And once you've had cancer I suppose you always hope that there isn't a little bit floating around in there because you hear ... (Story continues uninterrupted for several minutes.)

Here the black hole of denial is gently and slowly entered with a touch of distancing and humor.

During the interview the interviewer is taking brief notes, referred to as "field jottings" by Bernard (1988). These notes include observations about the respondent (e.g., nervous or evasive), the surroundings (e.g., temperature, noise, distractions), and about the interview itself (e.g., the number of interruptions, changes in type of communication). Notes to facilitate remembering any key terms and names are also kept.

When the official interview is over and the tape recorder is turned off, it is important to linger for 5-15 minutes of postinterview contact. This is the time for closing small talk, which sets a tone of empowerment and good relations. It is also an opportunity to elicit the respondent's impressions of the interview and to be alert for the unguarded moment when new information is revealed (Gordon, 1975). And say thank-you!

THE FINAL SCRIPT:
EVALUATION AND TRANSCRIPTION

Before transcription an interview needs to be evaluated for quality and then transcribed only if acceptable. This evaluation process, as discussed by Whyte (1984), is to ensure the sound quality of the tape, the overall quality of the interview as it relates to the information the interviewer was trying to obtain, and the assessment of ulterior motives and distortions. This screening prevents unnecessary transcription expense. The actual transcription will take approximately 4 to 6 hours for every 1 hour of interview.

## Conclusions

The creative semistructured depth interview is an entranceway to narrative understanding. It balances intimacy and distance, which opens the way to understanding how particular individuals arrive at the cognitions, emotions, and values they presently hold. We have presented one particular type of depth interview, the Long Interview, and illustrated its use as a data collection tool in a study about pain. The analysis of these data is presented in Chapter 17. This artificial separation of data collection and data analysis is unfortunate, since in actual field research both these processes occur in circular iterative fashion. Interviews are analyzed as they are collected, and modifications in the guide or changes in the sampling strategy are made before the next series of interviews. The understanding of "truth" emerges within the research process, not in a significance level at the end.

## References

Barnhouse, A. H., Kilodychuk, G. R., Pankratz, C., & Olinger, D. A. (1988). Evaluation of acute pain: A comparison of patient and nurse perspectives. *Journal of Nursing Quality Assurance, 2,* 54-63.

Bernard, H. R. (1988). *Research methods in cultural anthropology.* Newbury Park, CA: Sage.

Blake, R. L., & Bertuso, D. D. (1988). The life space drawing as a measure of social relationships. *Family Medicine, 20,* 295-297.

Briggs, C. D. (1986). *Learning how to ask.* Cambridge: Cambridge University Press.

Denzin, N. K. (1989a). *Interpretive interactionism.* Newbury Park, CA: Sage.

Denzin, N. K. (1989b). *Interpretive biography.* Newbury Park, CA: Sage.

Diamond, E. L., & Grauer, K. (1986). The physician's reaction to patients with chronic pain. *American Family Physician, 34,* 117-122.

Douglas, J. D. (1985). *Creative interviewing.* Beverly Hills, CA: Sage.

Dunn, W. R., & Hamilton, D. D. (1986). The critical incident technique: A brief guide. *Medical Teacher, 8,* 207-215.

Ellen, R. F. (1984). *Ethnographic research: A guide to general conduct.* New York: Academic Press.

Fagerhaugh, S. Y., & Strauss, A. (1977). *Politics of pain management: Staff-patient interaction.* Menlo Park, CA: Addison-Wesley.

Fields, H. L. (1987). *Pain.* New York: McGraw-Hill.

Frank, A. J. M., Moll, J. M. H., & Hurt, J. F. (1982). A comparison of three ways of measuring pain. *Rheumatology and Rehabilitation, 21,* 211-217.

Gordon, R. L. (1975). *Interviewing: Strategy, techniques and tactics.* Homewood, IL: Dorsey.

Gottlieb, M. (1986). *Interview.* New York: Longman.

Hilbert, R. A. (1984). The acultural dimensions of chronic pain: Flawed reality construction and the problem of meaning. *Social Problems, 31,* 365-378.

Kirk, J., & Miller, M. L. (1986). *Reliability and validity in qualitative research.* Beverly Hills, CA: Sage.

Kleinman, A., & Good, B. (Eds.). (1985). *Culture and depression: Studies in the anthropology and cross-cultural psychiatry of affect and disorder.* Berkeley: University of California Press.

Kotarba, J., & Seidel, J. (1984). Managing the problem pain patient: Compliance or social control. *Social Science and Medicine, 19,* 1393-1400.

McCracken, G. (1988). *The Long Interview.* Beverly Hills, CA: Sage.

McGoldrick, M., & Gerson, R. (1985). *Genograms in family assessment.* New York: Norton.

Merton, R. K., Fiske, M., & Kendall, P. L. (1956). *The focused interview: A manual of problems and procedures.* Glencoe, IL: Free Press.

Mishler, E. G. (1986). *Research interviewing.* Cambridge, MA: Harvard University Press.

Patton, M. Q. (1987). *How to use qualitative methods in evaluation.* Beverly Hills, CA: Sage.

Pelto, P. J., & Pelto, G. H. (1978). *Anthropological research: The structure of inquiry* (2nd ed.). Cambridge: Cambridge University Press.

Perry, S. W. (1985). Irrational attitudes towards addicts and narcotics. *Bulletin of the New York Academy of Medicine, 61,* 706-723.

Sacks, H., Schegloff, E. A., & Jefferson, G. (1974). A systematics for organization of turntaking for conversation. *Language, 50,* 696-735.

Schatzman, L., & Strauss, A. L. (1973). *Field research: Strategies for a natural sociology.* Englewood Cliffs, NJ: Prentice-Hall.

Spradley, J. P. (1979). *The ethnographic interview.* New York: Holt, Reinhart & Winston.

Watson, L. C., & Watson-Franke, M. (1985). *Interpreting life histories.* New Brunswick, NJ: Rutgers University Press.

Weller, S. C., & Romney, A. K. (1988). *Systematic data collection.* Beverly Hills, CA: Sage.

Whyte, W. F. (1984). *Learning from the field: A guide from experience.* Beverly Hills, CA: Sage.

# PART FIVE

## TOOLS FOR ANALYSIS

# 17 The Analysis of Narratives From a Long Interview

BENJAMIN F. CRABTREE
WILLIAM L. MILLER

Uncertainty, suffering, conflicting expectations, illness experiences, choices, and pattern recognition: These are a few of the many issues that primary care providers and researchers wish to understand. These and similar areas of concern have sparked an increase in interest in techniques for analyzing such text-based data as observational field notes and interview transcripts. This chapter will present in detail a constant comparative method for narrative analysis that can yield taxonomies, themes and theses, and general grounded theory. It will also briefly review alternative styles of analysis and position all of these in the larger context of a typology of research methods.

When a patient and doctor meet in a small alcohol-redolent room behind a closed door, much complex process occurs prior to any outcome measures. Attempts to generate clinically useful questions about this process have led to a growing awareness that primary care research cannot rely solely on an epidemiological perspective. It is not that epidemiological approaches are inherently flawed; rather that they are inappropriately applied when the research questions still require the identification and description of poorly understood substantive phenomena. Concerns about this deficit, and a recognition that additional research paradigms may prove helpful, have appeared recently in the primary care literature (Candib, 1988; Engel, 1977, 1987; Freymann, 1989; Kuzel, 1986; Phillips, 1988; Ruane, 1988) and have been voiced at conferences and national meetings (Blake, Broadhead, Feinstein, & Miller, 1989; Irby, 1988; McWhinney, 1989). Primary care researchers are now cognizant of a growing array of alternative methods, several of which are presented in this book (Focus Groups and the Long Interview).

Many fieldwork methods rely on field notes from observations or interviews (see Chapter 16) and often involve text analysis. Unfortunately, specific descriptions of how actually to use these techniques remain scarce in the primary care literature. In the remainder of this chapter we will investigate the use of one fieldwork method, the Long Interview (McCracken, 1988), with primary attention on the analysis of interview transcripts. In order to provide a context for the Long Interview, we will first briefly review a typology of methods available for primary care researchers and then overview general approaches to text analysis.

## A Typology of Primary Care Research Methods

The overwhelming bulk of published primary care research is based on observational epidemiologic methods. This is much too narrow a methodological vision, as it ignores a rich tradition of fieldwork, nonreactive, and other survey methods. Scientific knowing begins with the identification of the phenomena that compose the substantive world and proceeds to describe those phenomena both systemically and reductionistically. Once described, associations and differences between the phenomena are discovered and explanatory theories generated. These associations and theories then are tested in an effort to demonstrate causality and to confirm their truth value and predictive value. Finally, scientific knowing seeks to change and control the substantive world.

For example, primary care clinicians and researchers identify the phenomenal units that comprise "pain," and describe its content and context. They proceed to link this described "hand, back, and hip pain" to such other phenomena as "red eyes, stooped posture, fatigue, and abandonment by husband" and to generate a theory to explain the associations. Measurement tools are developed, hypotheses tested, and predictions confirmed. Finally, treatment strategies are developed and evaluated.

Each of these levels of inquiry asks different questions, each better answered by different methods. Similarly each method has its own associated design, sampling, data collection, data analysis, outcome, and reporting options. Which specific method is more appropriate depends not only on the conceptual level of inquiry but also on the desired outcome measures, the acceptable underlying paradigmatic assumptions, and the orientation of the researcher.

The Long Interview, as described by McCracken (1988), is one type of depth interview technique within the fieldwork research style. The fieldwork style methods all can be used from three different perspectives:

ethnographic, clinical, and collaborative. These three perspectives are most easily distinguished by the primary source of the research agenda. The ethnographic perspective is field research based on the researcher's question of interest; the clinical perspective is field research based on a client's (such as a hospital administrator's) question of interest; and the collaborative perspective is driven by the "subject's" research question. Clinical fieldwork methods such as the Long Interview originally were developed in support of marketing research interest.

## Approaches to Text Analysis

In the Long Interview, McCracken proposes an analytic sequence similar to the constant comparative method used by Glaser and Strauss (1968). Selected utterances are identified and highlighted in the transcripts, and observations are recorded about these segments. Following comparison of these observations, themes and theses are formulated. This approach to text analysis "edits" segments of the data that seem relevant and uses these as the basis for interpretation.

Other analytic styles could also be used in the analysis of Long Interview data. In our review of the available literature on approaches to text analysis, we have been able to distinguish four general styles falling on a continuum from deductive to inductive: (a) manifest content analysis, in which key words or phrases are quantitatively tallied (Mostyn, 1985; Weber, 1985); (b) approaching the data with highly structured a priori codebooks (Bee & Crabtree, 1992; Miles & Huberman, 1984); (c) an editing approach, in which the researcher explicitly and systematically reduces and reassembles the data (McCracken, 1988; Mishler, 1986; Spradley, 1979; Werner & Schoepfle, 1987a, 1987b); and (d) an immersion/crystallization approach, in which the interpreter becomes immersed in the text and crystallizes its core understanding (Bleicher, 1980; Fetterman, 1989; Rabinow & Sullivan, 1979). Within each of these styles is considerable variation, depending on the data, the research focus, and the disciplinary tradition.

Manifest content analysis (also referred to as basic content analysis) is intended to describe the surface "what" of textual material. (The other three analytic styles all address the "why" or intent of the generators of the text.) It is initiated with a priori or deductive determination of such units as words, sentences, themes, or descriptive phrases. Categories and scoring systems are set up; the text is coded; and words, theme regularities, and scores are tallied. Such cultural products as songs and poems, nonverbal communications, dreams, propaganda, and patient-therapist interactions are examples of text addressed by manifest content analysis.

In summary this analytic style is deductive, explicitly systematic, highly reliable, and provides accurate superficial descriptions.

A second analytic style is the use of templates to identify latent content, meaning, and structure. Prior to text analysis, a codebook is developed that identifies and defines the themes, language, domains, categories, and events of interest, based on a review of the literature and of the researcher's preconceived ideas. This codebook then is applied to the text, and the coded text is analyzed, using data display tables and matrices that make explicit the interpretative data reductions. Miles and Huberman (1984) have described this analytic style in detail. Multidimensional scaling, an analytic technique used on ethnoscience pile sort data, is an example of a more quantitative approach that uses terms elicited from this analytic style (Romney, Shepard, & Nerlove, 1972; Weller & Romney, 1988). The template style, in short, is essentially deductive, explicitly systematic, fairly reliable, and addresses the latent content.

The immersion/crystallization style, on the other hand, is inductive, intuitive, and intensely data-driven. With this approach the literature often is not reviewed until after analysis has begun. The researcher immerses her- or himself into the text and, from this fresh encounter with the narrative, a holistic understanding of the text is crystallized. Specific techniques using this style include existential truth analysis (Douglas & Johnson, 1977) and heuristic research (Moustakas, 1990). The immersion/crystallization style is the most inductive, least explicit, and least reliable but is often quite valid and is frequently the source of new insights and discoveries.

The editing style is the most commonly used and has many variations based on the specific fieldwork method employed. What distinguishes this style of analysis is its inductive but explicitly cut-and-paste aspects. All editing techniques start with the data and then systematically arrange, code, rearrange, and recode them until interpretation is complete. This is the style characteristic of ethnoscientific structural analysis (Werner & Schoepfle, 1987a, 1987b), while phenomenology uses hermeneutic (Packer & Addison, 1989; Rabinow & Sullivan, 1979) and semiotic analytic techniques (Manning, 1987). The editing style reveals the deep "why" content of narrative text inductively but systematically with fair reliability.

## Analysis of Long Interview Narratives

Data analysis, referred to by McCracken as the discovery of analytic categories, is a series of analysis stages that progressively become more abstract and interpretive. The first stage of this type of analysis (called the *constant comparative method*) begins with each member of the research team identifying key utterances in the text and making interpretive notations about them in the margins. The notations or observations (not the original text itself) of each interpreter are then systematically compared and expanded until salient themes emerge. Summarized themes for each respondent are compared with other respondents' themes until broader themes, or theses, are discovered and described.

We use an administered research approach that utilizes a team of researchers rather than an individual. We believe this approach is more feasible given the time constraints of many academic researchers. In addition, by having an interdisciplinary team, the analysis is strengthened greatly by the diversity of perspectives and by the improved ability to identify researcher biases that influence and direct the interpretation. The value of this administered approach becomes more apparent in the analysis presented below.

In the remainder of this chapter we illustrate the narrative analysis approach proposed by McCracken in the Long Interview, using transcribed interviews from a study comparing and contrasting physician and patient perceptions of pain and pain management (see Chapter 16). This study was conceived to identify and describe physician and patient experiences and understanding of pain and its management. We hope to develop comparative pain taxonomies and to discover common and differentiating themes.

The original anomaly leading to this research was the observation that physicians rarely utilize optimal pain management strategies despite numerous studies chiding them for underutilization of pain medications (e.g., see Bond, 1983; Hammond, 1979; Marks & Sachar, 1973; Morgan & Fleet, 1983). This chapter presents the analysis of one of the six physician-patient pairs that were interviewed. We first focus on the analysis of the physician transcript in a step-by-step description of the process in order to identify themes within a single interview. The process of comparing themes between different interviews then is illustrated by introducing a major theme of the patient's and using it to comparatively broaden the themes into theses and general hypotheses.

### Step 1: Utterance Identification and Making Observations

The first step of the analysis is to identify utterances or phrases in the transcript and to indicate what makes them noteworthy. Each of the researchers on the team independently reads the interview narrative and marks (using a highlighter) those phrases of the respondent that they feel are significant: for example, key terms, metaphors, interpretations, statements that suggest underlying assumptions and values, and immediate referents to the question or to analytic/cultural categories. Simultaneous with this *utterance identification* phase is *the making of observations*. For example, in the following paragraph from the physician transcript, the text in bold indicates utterances highlighted by one of the analysts:

> Well, it's I guess. . . **partly that has to be how I can relate to it. If somebody comes in, having, you know, slammed their finger in a door, that is something I can. . . I've done it in the past. Or if it's something I can imagine. . . then all I can do is base it on my own, um, level of pain.** And if it doesn't seem like it should be that bad, then sometimes I'm surprised at how much it bothers the person. Although I'm realizing more and more, when I'm in practice, that I have to, you know. . . . **everybody has different pain thresholds.** And you just can't, um. . . . what seems minimal to you. . . . it doesn't matter what it seems to. . . . what it would be, really, **because everybody's different. And so one person might stub their toe and not even notice, and the other person might need crutches' cause they stubbed their toe. And that's fine. That's just the way it is. You can't do anything about it, so. . .except accept it.**

Notations were made adjacent to each highlighted line of text describing why it was highlighted. For example, this analyst noted in the margin next to the first highlighted utterance:

**Experience of pain is key to it being believable (good or bad)**

Next to the last block of highlighted text, the notation was:

**Different perceptions are how it is (different thresholds)**

The other researchers in the team agreed with the first notation; however, one researcher had noted the following for the last block of highlighted text:

**Accepts that people have different tolerances of pain—has some kind of negative implication? Some people have minor pain but make a big deal.**

The initial notations can be thought of as interpretive observations made by each interviewer. At this stage it is important to limit each observation to its specific narrative context; that is, the researcher should not be trying to relate this utterance to any others. This is particularly difficult, since as researchers we are continually trying to abstract and seek closure. As in the practice of primary care, one must always beware of premature closure. Differences in the observations are resolved in the subsequent step of the analysis, when the researchers discuss matters as a group.

### Step 2: Expansion of Observations

Next, all members of the team confer and discuss the interview in detail, going virtually line by line to reach a consensus on which text should be highlighted and whether the marginal notations are justified. In the example presented above, the last block of highlighted text resulted in a protracted discussion: one notation emphasizing only that people have different thresholds, the other that this makes a negative statement about patients. While not a major disagreement, these differences in interpretation must be negotiated on the basis of data provided in the text or in the interview field notes. In this case the group consensus was that the highlighted utterance could be justifiably interpreted as:

**Value conflict: 1. My self disvalues overestimation; 2. My doctor self disvalues not believing patient's pain is real, i.e., I'm uncomfortable, so just accept it.**

This interpretation generated a hypothesis about the physician placing a negative value on certain patients. This hypothesis now needs to be checked against the remainder of the text or at a follow-up interview. Thus the implications and possibilities of each observation are expanded on by the group. This *expansion of observation* process frequently suggests linkages between several observations as shown in the following selection of text taken from later in the interview:

It kind of **depends on how well I know them.** I really am hesitant to give anyone who I don't know very well, **a first-time patient** who comes in complaining of migraines, um, that type of pain med. And I tell them that. That I really don't know them, and I don't know their past history, and **it's just generally not my practice to do that until I've established a relationship with them.** Because if I do give them something like Demerol or whatever, **I'm really nagging about, "You can't take this all the time, it's addictive." And ALL the time, I'm bringing up how we're going to have to cut this out.** And I eventually do. (Laughs.) So, I'm pretty true to my word in terms of getting them off. **And I've lost a fair amount of patients because of that, you know. They don't like that. So, um, I try to set limits in terms of taking those types of pain meds.**

In this paragraph the value conflict noted earlier is revealed again, giving support to the observations and hypothesis noted above. This conflict, however, can also be understood as a conflict between the person-centered approach expected of a family physician and the need to control addiction. This latter need appears to have a higher priority than the person—even to the extent that patients become expendable. This is suggestive evidence of a distinction between "professional pain" and "personal pain" for this particular physician. This interpretation leads us to the next step.

### Step 3: Comparison of Observations

After the transcript is reviewed by the group, the expanded observations are compared systematically, looking for organizing concepts, contradictions, and similarities. In this *comparison of observation* phase the actual narrative is referred to only to confirm or challenge the refined observations. This step is facilitated by editing the transcript so that only the highlighted utterances remain and then by typing observations from the text margins into a separate file. From these reduced data, key organizing concepts can be identified. Several of the key organizing concepts for this physician include addiction, patient control, value conflict, and explanation of cause. These concepts or categories become headings, which are not necessarily mutually exclusive. The observations are sorted into one or more of these categories. For example, the expanded observation negotiated above would fall into the categories of patient control, as well as value conflict. The selected utterances that produced the observations are identified and matched with the pertinent observation. These are organized into a written summary suggesting "a field of patterns and themes." This summary is equivalent to a research codebook and could be used to code text as in the a priori codebook approach noted earlier.

### Step 4: Theme Development

The written summary leads to *theme development*, the stage in which most data reduction and interpretation occur. All the complexities, apparent paradoxes, and detailed richness of the text are hierarchically organized into summary arrays of themes that answer the research question as it relates to each individual respondent. In this phase it is possible to utilize the highlighted utterances, as well as the categorized observations. Possible themes are checked against other categories of selected utterances and observations until this respondent's understanding of pain is revealed in a manner consistent with all available text. A major theme from this physician's interview was the conflict between personal beliefs and experiences about pain and pain management, and those beliefs internalized as a medical student and family medicine resident. A real dilemma exists between the belief that the doctor should listen to the patient, understand the holistic context, and negotiate treatment strategies, versus the absolute necessity to avoid addiction and to enforce this view even to the extent that the patient is driven from the practice. This physician wishes patients would be more like herself, that is, tolerate pain and use medications only when "really necessary."

*Step 5: Comparison of*
*Interview Themes*

Once themes have been identified for each respondent, *comparison of different interview themes* are made. The goal is to compare and contrast the cultural categories and themes of the individual interviews and to transform them into analytic categories or theses. These then can be generalized to an appropriate theory. In our research this generalization would expand the analysis beyond the models and themes of individual physicians, into both a comparison of models and themes within each physician-patient pair, and eventually a comparison of the different physician-patient pairs. To illustrate this process it is necessary to summarize briefly the key themes for the patient in this first physician-patient pair.

The same text analysis style described above was applied to the transcript generated by the patient. One of the main themes for this individual is the importance of maintaining control and understanding why pain exists. For her, understanding helps in the ability to "handle the pain"; it relieves the worry and allows her to live with the pain and not to rely on drugs that merely cover it up. She also feels that "pain babies" are unable to distinguish between real pain and not real pain; these persons overutilize doctors and medications, thus influencing the primary role of the doctor—that of helping the patient understand. Unfortunately the doctor seldom takes the time to listen to the patient (the result of "pain babies" and an overriding concern with making money). The doctor also tends not to explain what is causing the pain and has a tendency to "use drugs and not time." Thus the core theme for this patient—staying in control in her everyday life in an almost heroic manner—has related subthemes, including the "doctor as sacred friend" and "real pain versus imaginary pain." These subthemes are also associated with consultation and management patterns for this individual.

Comparison of themes for this pair reveals some striking similarities between patient and doctor. Both have strong views about the need for the former to participate actively in the relationship and to understand the cause of pain. Both also minimize pain and the need for medication. By comparing the themes of each we begin to formulate an analytic thesis, which states that the physician and patient both have personal visions of pain derived from personal experience, and which support their personal identities. Both also have a professional vision of pain, but here these visions are from different sources. The physician learns from within the profession and uses this vision to support a professional identity, whereas the patient learns from contact with professionals and uses this vision to again support her personal identity. In summary, the physician has potentially conflicted identities, the patient harmonious identities. One hypothesis suggested by this thesis is that patient satisfaction with the doctor-patient relationship may be dependent on the doctor's using that model of pain (personal and professional) most complementary to the patient's model.

This thesis then is compared and contrasted with that found in other doctor-patient pairs from the study, thus *identifying* and *describing* some of the perceptions of both patients and physicians. These conclusions are generalizable to theory, and their transferability can be evaluated in other settings. Specifically the thesis proposed above lends possible support to the patient-centered approach developed by the Doctor-patient Communication Group of The University of Western Ontario, which proposes (and offers supporting evidence) that the physician should both perform differential diagnosis and understand the patient's illness experience and then negotiate a management plan (Bass et al., 1986; Brown, Weston, & Stewart, 1990; Levenstein et al., 1989; Stewart, Brown & Weston, 199; Weston, Brown, & Stewart, 1990). The preliminary thesis derived from our text analysis supports this theory and suggests that the physician can use his or her personal pain model to facilitate understanding of the patient's illness experience.

## Conclusions

When the goal of primary care research is the identification and description of poorly understood phenomena and the generation of hypotheses pertinent to the clinical setting, fieldwork research methods from the clinical perspective are very helpful. Most of these methodologies result in large quantities of text requiring analysis. We have presented one editing style approach for doing this text analysis. We concentrated on the analytic technique and have purposely not discussed verification tactics, since excellent reviews of these already exist (Kuzel

& Like, 1991; Lincoln & Guba, 1985). In the final analysis, trustworthiness is best tested in practice.

## References

Bass, M. J., Buck, C., Turner, L., Dickie, G., Pratt, G., & Robinson, H. C. (1986). The physician's actions and the outcome of illness in family practice. *Journal of Family Practice, 23*(1), 43-47.

Bee, R. L., & Crabtree, B. F. (1992). Using ethnograph in fieldnote management. In M. S. Boone & J. Wood (Eds.), *Computer applications in anthropology* (pp. 91-112). New York: Wadsworth.

Blake, R. L., Broadhead, W. E., Feinstein, A. R., & Miller, W. L. (1989, May). *Approaches to qualitative data.* Round table discussion at the 17th Annual Meeting of the North America Primary Care Research Group, Ottawa, Canada.

Bleicher, J. (1980). *Contemporary hermeneutics.* Boston: Routledge & Kegan Paul.

Bond, M. R. (1983). Patient's experience of pain. In N. E. Williams & H. Wilson (Eds.), *Pain and its management* (pp. 1-11). Oxford: Pergamon Press.

Brown, J. B., Weston, W. W., & Stewart, M. A. (1990). Patient-centred interviewing, part 2: Finding common ground. *Canadian Family Physician, 35,* 153-157.

Candib, L. M. (1988). Ways of knowing in family medicine: Contributions from a feminist perspective. *Family Medicine, 20*(2), 133-136.

Douglas, J. D., & Johnson, J. M. (Eds). (1977). *Existential sociology.* New York: Cambridge University Press.

Engel, G. L. (1977). The need for a new medical model: A challenge for biomedicine. *Science, 196,* 129-136.

Engel, G. L. (1987). Physician-scientists and scientific physicians: Resolving the humanism-science dichotomy. *American Journal of Medicine, 82,* 107-111.

Fetterman, D. M. (1989). *Ethnography step by step.* Newbury Park, CA: Sage

Freymann, J. G. (1989). The public's health care paradigm is shifting, medicine must swing with it. *Journal of General Internal Medicine, 4,* 313-319.

Glaser, B. G., & Strauss, A. L. (1968). *The discovery of grounded theory: Strategies for qualitative research.* London: Weidenfeld & Nicolson.

Hammond, D. (1979). Unnecessary suffering: Pain and the doctor-patient relationship. *Perspectives in Biology and Medicine, 23*(1), 153-161.

Irby, D. M. (1988, November). *Paradigms and revolutions: Medical education in transition.* Invited address to the Annual Conference for Generalists in Medical Education, Chicago.

Kuzel, A. J. (1986). Naturalistic inquiry: An appropriate model for family medicine. *Family Medicine, 18*(6), 369-374.

Kuzel, A. J., & Like, R. C. (1991). Standards of trustworthiness for qualitative studies in primary care. In P. G. Norton, M. Stewart, F. Tudiver, M. J. Bass, & E. V. Dunn (Eds.), *Primary care research: Traditional and innovative approaches* (pp. 138-158). Newbury Park, CA: Sage.

Levenstein, J. H., Brown, J. B., Weston, W. W., Stewart, M., McCracken, E. C., & McWhinney, I. (1989). Patient-centred clinical interviewing. In M. Stewart & D. Roter (Eds.), *Communicating with medical patients* (pp. 107-120). Newbury Park, CA: Sage.

Lincoln, Y. S., & Guba, E. G. (1985). *Naturalistic inquiry.* Beverly Hills, CA: Sage.

Manning, P. K. (1987). *Semiotics and fieldwork.* Newbury Park, CA: Sage.

Marks, R. M., & Sachar, E. J. (1973). Undertreatment of medical inpatients with narcotic analgesics. *Annals of Internal Medicine, 78*(2), 173-181.

McCracken, G. (1988). *The Long Interview.* Newbury Park, CA: Sage.

McWhinney, I. R. (1989, May). *An acquaintance with particulars.* Curtis B. Hames Research Award Lecture presented at the 22nd Annual Conference of the Society of Teachers of Family Medicine, Denver, Colorado.

Miles, M. B., & Huberman, A. M. (1984). *Qualitative data analysis.* Beverly Hills, CA: Sage.

Mishler, E. G. (1986). *Research interviewing.* Cambridge, MA: Harvard University Press.

Morgan, J. P., & Fleet, D. L. (1983). Opiophobia in the United States: The undertreatment of severe pain. In J. P. Morgan & D. V. Kagan (Eds.), *Society and medication: Conflicting signals for prescribers and patients* (pp. 313-325). Lexington, MA: Lexington.

Mostyn, B. (1985). The content analysis of qualitative research data: A dynamic approach. In M. Brenner, J. Brown, & D. Canter (Eds.), *The research interview: Uses and approaches* (pp. 115-145). New York: Academic Press.

Moustakas, C. (1990). *Heuristic research; Design, methodology, and applications.* Newbury Park, CA: Sage.

Packer, M. J., & Addison, R. B. (1989). *Entering the circle: Hermeneutic investigation in psychology.* Albany, NY: SUNY Press.

Phillips, T. J. (1988). Disciplines, specialties, and paradigms. *Journal of Family Practice, 27*(2), 139-141.

Rabinow, R., & Sullivan, W. M. (Eds.). (1979). *Interpretive social science.* Berkeley: University of California Press.

Romney, A. K., Shepard, R. N., & Nerlove, S. B. (Eds.). (1972). *Multidimensional scaling: Theory and applications in behavior sciences* (Vol. 2). New York: Seminar.

Ruane, T. J. (1988). Paradigms lost: A central dilemma for academic family practice. *Journal of Family Practice, 27*(2), 133-135.

Spradley, J. P. (1979). *The ethnographic interview.* New York: Holt, Reinhart & Winston.

Stewart, M. A., Brown, J. B., & Weston, W. W. (1990). Patient-centred interviewing, part 3: Five provocative questions. *Canadian Family Physician, 35*, 159-161.

Weber, R. (1985). *Basic content analysis.* Beverly Hills, CA: Sage.

Weller, S. C., & Romney, A. K. (1988). *Systematic data collection.* Newbury Park, CA: Sage.

Werner, O., & Schoepfle, G. M. (1987a). *Systematic fieldwork: Foundations of ethnography and interviewing.* Newbury Park, CA: Sage.

Werner, O., & Schoepfle, G. M. (1987b). *Systematic fieldwork: Ethnographic analysis and data management.* Newbury Park, CA: Sage.

Weston, W. W., Brown, J. B., & Stewart, M. A. (1990). Patient-centred interviewing, part 1: Understanding patients' experiences. *Canadian Family Physician, 35*, 147-151.

# 18 Statistical Packages for the Computer: Principles for Selection in Primary Care Research

PETER G. NORTON
EDMEE FRANSSEN
EARL V. DUNN

## Introduction

With the advent of the first computers—the mainframes of the 1950s and 1960s—it became possible to carry out accurate and relatively sophisticated tests on the large data bases that are generated in many primary care studies. These early machines, however, with their limited availability, could be used by only a small number of medical researchers and had very little impact on day-to-day primary care research. This all changed dramatically in the 1980s with the arrival of the personal computer. By the end of the decade most researchers either owned or had access to desktop machines that could easily outperform the mainframes of the early 1960s. The researcher also had available a large number of software packages at various levels of sophistication, which allowed the calculation of a number of statistics on most of the data collected in the course of a research effort. These packages ranged from programs on simple calculators to powerful mainframe packages such as SAS and SPSS.

Suddenly everyone was a statistician! Calculations such as ANOVA, MANOVA, discriminant analysis, and others more sophisticated still, became easy to carry out. Immediately two things happened. First, many researchers began using the most powerful (and usually the most complicated!) packages to do calculations that could more easily be done on a hand calculator or even with paper and pencil—in effect, using a shotgun to destroy a mosquito. Second, although the statistics used to interpret research results must be appropriate for the hypothesis and the type of data collected, most of the packages could calculate many statistics, so researchers often reported inappropriate and misleading results (Hofacker, 1983; Lew, 1985). This chapter looks at some of the issues related to the first topic: that of selecting appropriate and useful statistical and related software for primary care research needs.

To aid in this difficult task, we present basic principles in three areas—statistics, hardware, and statistical software packages—and discuss the qualities of various packages as they relate to these principles. The chapter should not be viewed as endorsing any particular software: The packages discussed were selected only because they illustrate our principles and are ones that have been employed by the authors. The available computer software changes daily, and the new versions of well-known programs can be very different from the previous versions. Be wary and skeptical! Interested readers are referred to an extensive review of statistical software carried out by *PC Magazine* (Goldstone, 1989), and to reviews of statistical packages for medical research by Chan and Portnoy (1988) and by Clochesy (1987).

## Statistics

PRINCIPLE 1. Only those trained and experienced in statistical calculations can make proper use of all the modules included in the more complex packages.

On your own, use only the simpler modules of complex packages. Only use those with which you have complete familiarity. It is important that you be well acquainted with any module that you use. If more sophisticated or unfamiliar analyses need to be done, get help or send the job out to someone with more expertise.

PRINCIPLE 2. Do not undertake a statistical analysis without consultation unless you understand the basic principles and assumptions that underlie it.

Statistical packages, particularly menu-driven ones, can look deceptively simple and can appear to be working well while producing absurdities. This appearance is rarely because of a flaw in the program: More commonly the analysis being attempted is inappropriate for the type of data (Brown & Beck, 1988a, b, c, 1989a, b; Rodbard, Cole, & Munson, 1984). One approach to avoiding this problem is to use one of several available systems programmed to check that only appropriate statistics are employed. Some of these systems are of the paper-or-pencil type (for example, Andrews, Klem, Davidson, O'Malley, & Rodgers, 1981; Brown & Beck,

1988a, b, c, 1989a, b; Graziano & Paulin, 1989). Some packages are even computer-driven, such as Statistical Navigator and the program developed by Blum (1986). Unfortunately, to use such systems effectively, one must be something of an expert, able to answer rather complicated questions concerning the type of data and the underlying assumptions. Again, always consult a statistician when needed!

## Hardware

PRINCIPLE 3. Do not underestimate your needs.

Many hardware decisions need to be made when purchasing a system: Macintosh versus IBM; memory size; speed; and types of disk drive, monitor, printer, and other interfaces. All these are important, but the main thing to remember is that computer technology is changing at a very rapid rate and will continue to do so. Computers come in nearly as many varieties as do cars, and picking the right one is never easy. Six months from now the one you have chosen may not meet your needs. Make certain, therefore, that the machine you get can be upgraded easily and without too much cost. Do not scrimp on your memory and disk needs. Consider the basic programs you will use (complex programs such as SAS take up to 20 megabytes); the size of your data set; and whether you will be doing large sorts or other analyses that require data to be held in memory or in a "scratch" file, as this may triple the amount of space you need. For example, sorting a 1-megabyte DBASE III file may require nearly 3 megabytes of free space.

Luckily most good computers will accomplish all the needs of most researchers with reasonable performance and without any difficulties. If you need help in deciding what to purchase, talk to someone you trust. An understanding of the world of computer technology and availability is beyond most researchers, while salespeople do not usually understand the researcher's needs and are often unintentionally misleading.

## Statistical Software Packages

PRINCIPLE 4. For data entry, choose a system that will produce files that can be used by all the different software packages that you might employ. Within this constraint, choose the method that is most familiar to you and to the person who will be entering the data, and that will allow the maximum flexibility for error checking, handling missing data, and data manipulation.

Once raw data have been collected, one of the first tasks facing the researcher is entering them into the computer and performing any necessary pre-analysis manipulations. While many statistical packages can handle these functions adequately, most are not specifically designed for this aspect of research. Accordingly, whenever data are entered using one package, the files that result may not be usable by or easily transferred to a different package.

An ideal data entry system would be compatible with most statistical packages; allow automatic error checking on entry; have a short learning curve; and have the capacity for easy and powerful data manipulation, enabling one to join, manipulate, sort, transpose, or partition and split data sets quickly, accurately, and easily. An error-checking feature is especially important, since even a good data entry person can have up to a 2-3% error rate.

Look carefully at a package's ability to handle missing data. In the real world of research, this situation will occur often and must be handled easily and correctly (Albridge et al., 1988). Loss of data or the conversion of missing data to inappropriate values is common. For example, in DBASE II and III, if the data are manipulated (e.g., sorted) or exported to another program such as SAS, any missing data are converted to a value of 0. Thus, to avoid this conversion, it is necessary to use a dummy value (9 for example) when entering data into the DBASE program and then to convert this value after the manipulation is complete.

One particular problem in data manipulation deserves to be mentioned: data on time and dates. For storage and manipulation, many programs convert dates to a number that is the number of days after a specific date, for example, January 1, 1900. Know what your program does. How does the package handle date, time, and other similar variables? Appropriate storage of these types of variables can save much time and effort.

Often it is helpful to use one package for data entry and then transfer the data set to a statistical package. For entry we have usually elected to use either DBASE or LOTUS, for several reasons. Error checking can be easily built in with both programs; they are well known to most of the clerks who do our data entry; in the case of DBASE it is relatively easy to construct a menu-driven interface for data entry; both programs allow considerable flexibility in data manipulation; and many statistical packages can read and input directly from these packages.

One problem that long plagued us and others (Turley, 1989) had to do with the translation of files from one data entry program into a statistical program. Many of these problems have recently been solved with the arrival of DBMS/COPY, a program that can translate files between more than 75 data bases, spreadsheets, and statistical packages. It is easy to

e and almost, although not quite, solves many of the problems related
data entry and manipulation. With this program, data can be entered
ing LOTUS or DBASE and easily transferred to most statistical pro-
ams without any major problems arising over missing data or date
riables. One significant problem that should be noted, however, is that
quently an early version of a program will not read the data from a later
rsion of the same program, and here DMBS/COPY cannot always help.
you are exchanging data with a colleague using the same package and
e of you purchases an update, be careful!

INCIPLE 5. Carefully examine the interface of any package you are con-
nplating, and make certain you are comfortable with it. Some command-
e-driven packages involve complicated programming languages that
difficult to learn.

Some programs use a language that may already be familiar to you
m another program (some statistical packages use a version of BASIC,
example), and this common language can save a lot of headaches. If
u cannot or prefer not to use a mouse, then probably a program devel-
ed to use a mouse interface is not for you.

A poorly designed interface will require you to program the same
ps repeatedly; a well-designed interface allows you to do a task once
d then automate the procedure for future use. This feature saves time
d reduces the likelihood of errors in data manipulation. This automa-
n can be done in several ways, including learned macros and saved
mmand programs. Increasingly the newer packages have "assist"
ograms that will help you through most of the modules within the
ogram.

INCIPLE 6. The graphical capabilities of a statistical program are likely
be important. Graphs can help you understand your own data and
ll be used when you present to others. Choose a program that incor-
rates a reasonable graphics interface and that is compatible with other
ograms you may use. Also remember that the quality of your graphics
dependent on your printer.

Graphics are becoming one of the important features of the personal
mputer statistical packages: The ability to produce well-labeled, an-
tated graphs of many types directly from raw data enhances the
efulness and understandability of the results. For purposes of presen-
ion and publication, the production of graphic material is of utmost
portance. If you use a laser printer or programs such as Lotus Freelance
s, Harvard Graphics, or Polaroid Palette, be sure you can transfer
her your data or the completed graphs from the statistical package to
other utility package without too many hassles.

PRINCIPLE 7. Statistical packages are limited by the size of the data that can be analyzed. If you must analyze a very large data set on a si occasion, it probably should be sent out to a consultant for analysis general it is wise to limit the size of a data set to 80% of the maxim that your program will allow.

In an ideal world every statistical package would be able to han every data set. This is not always so: The size of data sets is limite most cases. The restrictions may apply to the number of variables, number of observations, both, or to the amount of free space to wl you can save a file. In our experience, when the data set approaches t of the maximum size available, errors begin to creep in: for exam data are transformed, or missing data are discarded.

PRINCIPLE 8. At times you will need help with the mechanics of program no matter how often you use it or how comfortable you feel v it. Ascertain whether the documentation and manuals are clear and un standable, and consider the availability of online help menus. When s ware is licensed through a large institution such as a university, help a be available at that source.

None of us knows it all. Frequently information is needed about program or the statistic that is being calculated. Many program man are weighty tomes in which it is hard to find things and that are o hard to understand. Most of the newer programs have online hel assist facilities, both for the program and for some of the statistics. I easy are these to use, and how helpful are they? Does the package w you when the test being done may be inaccurate or inappropriate? last can be a useful feature, expecially for an inexperienced user. Pi program with a good help facility, and then pay attention to any war or error message you might get!

PRINCIPLE 9. Statistical packages come in various levels of comple and with many different statistical computations. Choose the sma and simplest program that meets most of your present and future ne (At a minimum a good program should include all modules neede conduct basic analysis; for example, descriptive statistics, correlatic

Descriptive analysis is the first step in most primary care projects serves to identify possible erroneous data for verification and to un stand them for further analysis. All good packages should have a sir method to produce descriptive and other simple analyses without etitious and cumbersome programming.

Programs can be divided into three levels of sophistication: those produce simple descriptive data, those that carry out analyses of s data sets, and those that can do powerful analyses. The first, unless know a good programmer, can be used only to do the simple descrip of your data and some minimal analysis such as regression, but for most of us they serve a spreadsheet or data base function. The second type is programs such as Mystat, statistical programs that can carry out the more commonly used statistics on smaller data sets. They are relatively inexpensive and simple to use and will serve the needs of many primary care researchers. The third level type is large and very sophisticated programs, such as SYSTAT, SPSS, and SAS. These are less user-friendly but will do most of the analysis that a primary care researcher might ever need. Analyze your needs, and then pick the package or packages suited to them.

## Conclusions

The principles described above will help guide readers in the selection of the statistical packages that will best serve their needs. The world of personal computer software is changing constantly, especially in the field of statistics, in which needs and expertise vary so greatly between projects and researchers that it is difficult to define a "best" package, unlike data base, spreadsheet, or word processing programs, for which standards have been set. Thus be ready to select a package that will best meet your current needs, taking into consideration the near future and the possibility of upgrading both the hardware and software. It is hoped that the guidelines here will help the reader make the best possible decision in an unsettled domain.

## References

Albridge, K. M., Standish, J., & Fries, J. F. (1988). Hierarchical time-oriented approaches to missing data interference. *Computers in Biomedical Research, 21*(4), 349-366.

Andrews, F. M., Klem, L., Davidson, T. N., O'Malley, P. M., & Rodgers, W. L. (1981). *A guide for selecting statistical techniques for analyzing social science data.* Ann Arbor: University of Michigan, Institute for Social Research.

Blum, R. L. (1986). Computer-assisted design of study using routine clinical data. Analyzing the association of Prednisone and cholesterol. *Annals of Internal Medicine, 104*(6), 858-868.

Brown, R. A., & Beck, J. S. (1988a). Statistics on microcomputers: A non-algebraic guide to the appropriate use of statistical packages in biomedical research and pathology laboratory practice. A series of six articles. 1. Data handling and preliminary analysis. *Journal of Clinical Pathology, 41*(10), 1033-1038.

Brown, R. A., & Beck, J. S. (1988b). Statistics on microcomputers: A non-algebraic guide to the appropriate use of statistical packages in biomedical research and pathology laboratory practice. A series of six articles. 2. Confidence intervals and significance tests. *Journal of Clinical Pathology, 41*(11), 1148-1154.

Brown, R. A., & Beck, J. S. (1988c). Statistics on microcomputers: A non-algebraic guide to the appropriate use of statistical packages in biomedical research and pathology laboratory practice. A series of six articles. 3. Analysis of variance and distribution-free methods. *Journal of Clinical Pathology, 41*(12), 1256-1262.

Brown, R. A., & Beck, J. S. (1989a). Statistics on microcomputers: A non-algebraic guide to the appropriate use of statistical packages in biomedical research and pathology laboratory practice. A series of six articles. 4. Correlation and regression. *Journal of Clinical Pathology, 42*(1), 4-12.

Brown, R. A., & Beck, J. S. (1989b). Statistics on microcomputers: A non-algebraic guide to the appropriate use of statistical packages in biomedical research and pathology laboratory practice. A series of six articles. 5. Analysis of categorical data. *Journal of Clinical Pathology, 42*(2), 117-122.

Chan, L. S., & Portnoy, B. (1988). Evaluation of statistical packages for suitability for use by clinical investigators in medicine. *Computer Methods and Programs in Biomedicine, 27*(1), 83-94.

Clochesy, J. M. (1987). Computer use and nursing researcher: Statistical packages for microcomputers. *Western Journal of Nursing Research, 9*(1), 138-141.

Goldstone, R. (1989). Inside the world of numbers. *PC Magazine, 8*(5), 94-310.

Graziano, A. M., & Paulin, M. L. (1989). *Research methods: A process of inquiry.* New York: Harper & Row.

Hofacker, C. F. (1983). Abuse of statistical packages: The case of the general linear model. *American Journal of Physiology, 245*(3), 299-302.

Lew, R. A. (1985). Strategies for validation. *National Cancer Institute Monograph, 67,* 161-168.

Rodbard, D., Cole, B. R., & Munson, P. J. (1984). Development of a friendly, self-teaching, interactive statistical package for analysis of clinical research data: The BRIGHT STAT-PACK. *Journal of Medical Systems, 8*(3), 205-212.

Turley, J. P. (1989). Transferring data files between microcomputer statistical packages. *Nursing Research, 5,* 315-317.

# Appendix:
# Inventory of Psychosocial Measurement Instruments Useful in Primary Care

SCOTT H. FRANK

## Introduction

At the 1984 meeting of the Society of Teachers of Family Medicine (STFM) Task Force on Psychological Inventories in Family Medicine, the need was expressed for a compilation of psychosocial measurement tools that would be consistent with the special needs of family medicine. The list was to include instruments that could be used not only in clinical research but also in a patient care setting. Recognition of the busy nature of everyday practice mandated that the instruments be brief enough to administer with this constraint. While most of the instruments described here are short, I also have included some longer ones that are considered among the best in their areas, as well as a number of very long ones that have subscales.

In addition to the original reference for each instrument, when possible I have included a reference that describes its use in a family practice setting. The annotations represent comments from my personal use or evaluation to aid in decision making about which instruments to use.

An asterisk (*) represents instruments that I am aware have been used or developed in family medicine research.

AUTHOR'S NOTE: The inventory was created for the Society of Teachers of Family Medicine Task Force on Psychological Inventories in Family Medicine. The entire Department of Family Medicine at Case Western Reserve University School of Medicine contributed to the development of this compilation. In particular, I would like to thank Steve Zyzanski, PhD; Antonnette Graham, RN, MSW; and James Pretzer, PhD, for their support and expertise.

Many of the instruments are well established and have good data on reliability and validity. I have not hesitated, however, to include some that are still in the developmental stage in family practice settings.

Finally, this inventory is far from complete and does not claim to represent an exhaustive list. In each presentation new instruments have been added and more information has been provided for the annotations based on the experience of the participants.

This inventory contains 30 topics, and tests for each topic. The number of tests are as follows: depression, 12; anxiety, 10; stress response, 6; stress stimulus measures, 6; stress interaction measures, 6; support, 13; broad spectrum scales, 14; family function, 16; marital satisfaction, 11; communication, 3; health-risk behavior, 1; alcoholism, 6; tobacco dependency, 2; eating disorders, 2; somatization, 3; reason for visit, 1; coping, 10; self image/esteem, 7; personality, 5; functional status, 12; wellness, 3; pain, 4; locus of control, 1; patient satisfaction, 3; humanism, 1; sexual function, 6; anomy, 3; pediatric psychosocial tests, 5; geriatric psychosocial tests, 5; and mental status, 4.

## Depression

### BECK DEPRESSION INVENTORY (BDI)*

Item Number: 13 or 21
Item Format: 4-point ordered scale
Key References: Beck, A. T. & Beck, R. W. (1972). Screening depressed patients in family practice: A rapid technique. *Postgraduate Medicine, 52*(6), 81-85.
  Williamson H. A., & Williamson M. T. (1989). The Beck depression inventory: Normative data and problems with generalizability. *Family Medicine, 21,* 58-60.
Notes: Excellent for teaching about depression and for the clinical diagnosis of depression. A "gold standard" with a long track record, useful for validity testing of new instruments. Comparatively long; less effective at identifying depressed mood or lower levels of depression.

### ZUNG SELF-RATING DEPRESSION SCALE (SDS)*

Item Number: 20
Item Format: 4-point ordered scale
Key Reference: Zung, W. K. (1965). A self-rating depression scale. *Archives of General Psychiatry, 12,* 63-70.

Notes: Often used in primary care settings; probably the most studied instrument as a mental health screen in primary care. Relatively short, easy to understand, good patient acceptability. Long track record, many available comparisons. More diagnosis- than mood-oriented.

## DEPRESSION ADJECTIVE CHECKLIST (DACL)*

Item Number: 108
Key References: Lubin, B. (1965). Adjective checklists for measurement of depression. *Archives of General Psychiatry, 12*, 57-62.
  Davis T. C., Nathan R. G., Crouch M. A., et al. (1987). Screening depression in primary care: Back to the basics with a new tool. *Family Medicine, 19*, 200-202.
Notes: Recently compared with Beck Depression Inventory in a primary care setting and performed very well. Probably picks up a broader spectrum of depression.

## PROFILE OF MOOD STATES (POMS); DEPRESSION SCALE*

Item Number: 15
Item Format: 5-point ordered scale
Key References: McNair, D., Lorr, M., & Droppleman, L. (1971). *Profile of Mood States*. San Diego: Educational and Industrial Testing Service.
  Frank S. H., & Zyzanski S. J. (1988). Stress in the clinical setting: The brief encounter psychosocial instrument. *Journal of Family Practice, 26*, 533-539.
Notes: Excellent, brief, mood-oriented instrument with abundant comparison data available. Detects mild depression (depressed mood), as well as more serious depression. Can easily be "worked in" to an instrument assessing multiple problems.

## BRIEF SYMPTOM INVENTORY (BSI); DEPRESSION SCALE*

Item Number: 13
Item Format: 5-point ordered scale
Key Reference: Derogatis, L. R. (1977). *SCL-90-R administration, scoring, and procedures manual* (Vol. 1). Baltimore: Clinical Psychometric Research.
Notes: Excellent, brief, mood-oriented instrument with abundant comparison data available. Detects mild depression (depressed mood), as well as more serious depression. Can easily be "worked in" to an instrument assessing multiple problems. Derived from the SCLR 90.

## COSTELLO-COMREY DEPRESSION SCALE

Item Number: 14
Item Format: 9-point ordered scale
Key Reference: Costello, C. G., & Comrey, A. L. (1967). Scales for measuring
depression and anxiety. *The Journal of Psychology, 66*, 303-313.

## PERI SADNESS SCALE

Item Number: 4
Item Format: 5-point ordered scale
Key Reference: Social Psychiatry Research Unit. (1977, February). *The
psychiatric epidemiology research interview: A report on twenty-two scales,
Appendix I to the measurement of psychopathology in the community.* New
York: Columbia University Press. (mimeographed)

## PERI DESPAIR SCALE

Item Number: 6
Item Format: 5-point ordered scale
Key Reference: Social Psychiatry Research Unit. (1977, February). *The
psychiatric epidemiology research interview: A report on twenty-two scales,
Appendix I to the measurement of psychopathology in the community.* New
York: Columbia University Press. (mimeographed)

## LONELINESS SCALE

Item Number: 16
Item Format: 5-choice response scale
Key Reference: Francis, G. M. (1976). Loneliness: Measuring the abstract.
*International Journal of Nursing Studies, 13*, 153-160.

## HAMILTON DEPRESSION SCALE*

Item Number: 20
Item Format: Semistructured interview, rated on a scale of 1 to 4
Key References: Hamilton, M. (1967). Development of a rating scale for
primary depressive illness. *British Journal of Social Clinical Psychology,
6*, 278-296.
Beitman B. D., Basha I. M., Trombka L. H., et al. (1989). Pharmacotherapeutic treatment of panic disorder in patients presenting with
chest pain. *Journal of Family Practice, 28*, 177-180.

## DIAGNOSTIC INTERVIEW SCHEDULE (DIS);
## DEPRESSION SUBSCALE*

Key References: Robins L. N., Helzer J., Coughan J., et al. (1981). The National Institutes of Mental Health Diagnostic Interview Schedule: Its history, characteristics and validity. *Archives of General Psychiatry, 38*, 381-389.

Katon W., & Russo, J. (1989). Somatic symptoms and depression. *Journal of Family Practice, 29*, 65-69.

Cadoret R. J., & Widmer R. B. (1988). The development of depressive symptoms in the elderly following onset of severe physical illness. *Journal of Family Practice, 27*, 71-76.

Notes: The most important interview-format mental health screen. Designed to detect 16 different DSM-III-based diagnoses. Adaptation to self-administered format has just begun. Very long, but with useful subscales.


## CENTER FOR EPIDEMIOLOGIC STUDIES-DEPRESSION (CES-D)*

Item Number: 20

Key References: Radloff L. S. (1977). The CES-D Scale: A self-report depression scale for use in the general population. *Applied Psychological Measurement, 1*, 385-401.

Pascoe J. M., Ialongo N. S., Horn W. F., et al. (1988). The reliability and validity of the maternal social support index. *Family Medicine, 20*, 271-276.

Notes: Short, understandable, validated.


## Anxiety

### ZUNG SELF-RATING ANXIETY SCALE*

Item Number: 20

Item Format: 4-point ordered scale

Key Reference: Zung, W. K. (1971). A rating instrument for anxiety disorders. *Psychosomatics, 12*, 371-379.

Notes: Good companion piece to the more often used depression scale. Wide usage. Good patient acceptability.


### HAMILTON ANXIETY SCALE*

Item Number: 14

Item Format: Semistructured interview, rated on a scale of 1 to 4

Key References: Hamilton. M. (1969). Diagnosis and ratings of anxiety. *British Journal of Psychiatry, 3, 76-79.*
Beitman B. D., Basha I. M., Trombka L. H., et al. (1989). Pharmacotherapeutic treatment of panic disorder in patients presenting with chest pain. *Journal of Family Practice, 28, 177-180.*
Notes: One of the most commonly used anxiety scales.


## STATE TRAIT ANXIETY INDEX*

Item number: 40 (20 state; 20 trait)
Key References: Spielberger, C. D., Gorsuch, R. C., & Lushene, R. E. (1970). *Manual for the State-Trait Anxiety Inventory.* Palo Alto, CA: Consulting Psychologists.
Parker, J., & Rodney, W. (1986). Temperament and stress factors predictive of choosing to leave after one year of residency. *Family Medicine, 18, 308-310.*
Notes: Important conceptually, discriminating between "state" and "trait," a concept not often enough applied to other mental health issues. Excellent instrument, but a bit long.


## COSTELLO-COMREY ANXIETY SCALE

Item Number: 9
Item Format: 9-point ordered scale
Key Reference: Costello, C. G., & Comrey, A. L. (1967). Scales for measuring depression and anxiety, *Journal of Psychology. 66, 303-313.*


## GENERAL WELL-BEING ANXIETY SCALE

Item Number: 4
Item Format: 3 items with 6 item-specific categories; 1 item with 11 categories
Key Reference: Dupuy, H. J. (1972). The Psychological Section of the Current Health and Nutrition Examination Survey. *Proceedings of the Public Health Conference on Records and Statistics Meeting Jointly with the National Conference on Health Statistics* Washington, DC: National Center for Health Statistics.


## PERI ANXIETY SCALE

Item Number: 10
Item Format: 5-point ordered scale

Key Reference: Social Psychiatry Research Unit, (1977, February). *The Psychiatric Epidemiology Research Interview: A report on twenty-two scales, Appendix I to the measurement of psychopathology in the community* New York: Columbia University Press. (mimeographed)

## PERI DREAD SCALE

Item Number: 6
Item Format: 5-point ordered scale
Key Reference: Social Psychiatry Research Unit, (1977, February). *The Psychiatric Epidemiology Research Interview: A report on twenty-two scales, Appendix I to the measurement of psychopathology in the community.* New York: Columbia University Press. (mimeographed)

## PROFILE OF MOOD STATES (POMS); ANXIETY SCALE*

Item Number: 9
Item Format: 5-point ordered scale
Key References: McNair, D., Lorr, M., & Droppleman, L. (1971). *Profile of mood states.* San Diego: Educational and Industrial Testing Service.
Frank S. H., & Zyzanski S. J. (1988). Stress in the clinical setting: The brief encounter psychosocial instrument. *Journal of Family Practice, 26,* 533-539.
Notes: Excellent, brief, mood-oriented instrument with abundant comparison data available. Detects mild anxiety (anxious mood), as well as more serious depression. Can easily be "worked in" to an instrument assessing multiple problems.

## BRIEF SYMPTOM INVENTORY (BSI); ANXIETY SCALE*

Item Number: 10
Item Format: 5-point ordered scale
Key Reference: Derogatis, L. R. (1977). *SCL-90-R administration, scoring, and procedures manual* (Vol. 1). Baltimore: Clinical Psychometric Research.
Notes: Excellent, brief, mood-oriented instrument with abundant comparison data available. Detects mild anxiety (anxious mood), as well as more serious depression. Can easily be "worked in" to an instrument assessing multiple problems.

## INVENTORY OF GENERAL TRAIT ANXIOUSNESS

Item Number: 36
Item Format: 4 situations, 9 responses each

Key Reference: Endler, N. S., & Okada, M. (1975). A multidimensional measure of trait anxiety: The S-R Inventory of General Trait Anxiousness. *Journal of Consulting and Clinical Psychology, 43*, 319-329.

# Stress

## RESPONSE-ORIENTED MEASURES

### SYMPTOM RATING TEST

Item Number: 30
Key Reference: Kellner, R., & Sheffield, B. F. (1973). A self-rating scale of distress. *Psychological Medicine, 3*, 88-100.

### HOPKINS SYMPTOM INVENTORY CHECKLIST

Item Number: 58
Item Format: 4-point ordered scale
Subscales: Anxiety, depression, anger-hostility, obsessive-compulsive-phobic
Key Reference: Derogatis, L. R., Lipman, R. S., Rickels, K., Uhlenhuth, E. H., & Cou, L. (1974). The Hopkins Symptom Checklist (HSCL): A self-report symptom inventory. *Behavioral Science, 19*, 1-15.

### AFFECT BALANCE SCALE

Item Number: 10
Item Format: Yes/No
Key Reference: Bradburn, N. M. (1969). *The structure of psychological well-being.* Chicago: Aldine.
Notes: Short, useful instrument with reasonable results. Has stimulated more research in the area. Has components of "positive and negative affect."

### DEROGATIS AFFECT BALANCE SCALE

Item Number: 40
Item Format: 5-point ordered scale
Key Reference: Derogatis, L. R. (1975). *The Affect Balance Scale.* Baltimore: Clinical Psychometric Research.

### PSYCHOSOCIAL PROBLEMS INVENTORY

Item Number: 24

Item Format: Yes/No/Ooccasionally
Key Reference: Jacox, A., & Stewart, M. (1973). *Psychosocial contingencies of the pain experience.* Iowa City: University of Iowa.

## STIMULUS-ORIENTED MEASURES

### SOCIAL READJUSTMENT RATING SCALE*

Item Number: 42
Item Format: Yes/No (or scale)
Key Reference: Holmes, T, & Rahe, R. (1967). The Social Adjustment Rating Scale. *Journal of Psychosomatic Research, 11,* 213-218.
Notes: Historically important. The most commonly used "life change" measurement instrument. Most often used in 39- or 40-item format. Long.

### ATC SCHEDULE OF LIFE EVENTS*

Item Number: 12
Item Format: 5-point ordered scale
Key References: Rose, R. M., Jenkins, C. D., & Hurst, M. W. (1978). Health changes in air traffic controllers: A prospective study. *Psychosomatic Medicine, 40,* 142-165.
　　Frank S. H., & Zyzanski S. J. (1988). Stress in the clinical setting: The brief encounter psychosocial instrument. *Journal of Family Practice, 26,* 533-539.
Notes: Nice short-version life event scale. Gaining wider usage in family practice.

### DAILY HASSLES AND UPLIFTS SCALE

Item Number: 252 or 117
Item Format: 3-point scale
Key Reference: Kanner A. D., Coyne J. C., Schaefer C., & Lazarus, R. S. (1981). Comparison of two modes of stress measurement: Daily hassles and uplifts versus major life events. *Journal of Behavioral Medicine, 4,* 1-39
Notes: Important concept; quite long.

### OTOLOGIC SOURCES OF STRESS

Item Number: 69
Item Format: Open-ended scale

Key Reference: Ruznisky, S. A., & Thauberger, P. C. (1982). Incidents of reality: Sources of otological stress and concern. *Social Science Medicine, 16,* 1005-1011.
Notes: Nice concept, important reading, but unworkable as is. Have not seen any follow-up.


## OBSTETRICAL LIFE STRESS SCALE (1)

Item Number: 57
Item Format: Yes/No, then weighted response
Key Reference: Barnett, B. E. W., Hanna, B., & Parker, G. (1985). Life events scales for obstetrics groups. *Journal of Psychosomatic Medicine, 27,* 313-320


## THE STOKES-GORDON STRESS SCALE (SGSS)

Item Number: 104
Item Format: Checklist
Key Reference: Stokes S. A., & Gordon, S. E. (1988). Development of an instrument to measure stress in the older adult. *Nursing Research, 37*(1), 16-18


## INTERACTIONAL MEASURES


## BRIEF ENCOUNTER PSYCHOSOCIAL INSTRUMENT (BEPSI)

Item Number: 6
Item Format: 1 item opened-ended; 5 items scored on 5- or 10-point ordered scale
Key Reference: Frank, S. H., & Zyzanski, S. J. (1988). Stress in the clinical setting: The brief encounter psychosocial instrument. *Journal of Family Practice, 26,* 533-539.
Notes: Developed for use in primary care clinical and research settings. Meant to identify a spectrum of stress. Good psychometric properties for a short instrument. Helpful in teaching an interactive model of stress. Currently being field-tested with geriatric population.


## RATINGS OF STATEMENTS LIST

Item Number: 27
Item Format: 6-point scale
Key Reference: Van Dul, H., & Nagelkerke, N. (1980). Statistical discrimination of male myocardial infarction patients and healthy males by

means of a psychological test and a tracing of basic dimensions of the infarction personality. *Psychotherapy and Psychosomatics, 34,* 196-203.

## DEROGATIS STRESS PROFILE

Item Number: 77
Key Reference: Derogatis, L. R. (1980). *The Derogatis Stress Profile (DSP).* Baltimore: Clinical Psychometric Research.

## MAASTRICHT QUESTIONNAIRE

Item Number: 40 or 63
Item Format: Yes/No
Key Reference: Appels, A. (1980). Psychological prodromata of myocardial infarction and sudden death. *Psychotherapy and Psychosomatics, 35,* 213-223.

## THE PERSONAL (STRESS) INVENTORY

Item Number: 21
Item Format: 9-point scale, 5 subscales
Key Reference: Ireton, H. R. (1980). A personal inventory. *Journal of Family Practice, 11*(1), 137-140.
Notes: Developed in and for family practice. Good psychometric properties. Length is fine for research, possibly a bit long for patient care.

## THE PERCEIVED STRESS SCALE (PSS)

Item Number: 20
Item Format: 5-point scale
Key Reference: Cohen, S., Kamarck, T., & Mermelstein, R. (1983). A global measure of perceived stress. *Journal of Health and Social Behaviour, 24,* 385-396.
Notes: Nice instrument. Appears a bit longer than necessary but has excellent face validity.

## Support

## TANGIBLE ASSISTANCE*

Item Number: 1
Item Format: Multiple choice

Key Reference: Blake, R. L., & McKay, D. A. (1986). Single-item measure of
   social support as a predictor of morbidity. *Journal of Family Practice,*
   *22*(1), 82-84.
Notes: Amazing results for a single item. Very helpful concept clinically
   and in research.

## THE DUKE FUNCTIONAL SOCIAL SUPPORT SCALE*

Item Number: 8 to 14
Item Format: 5-point graphic scale
Subscales: Offers scores on "confidant support" and "affective support"
Key Reference: Broadhead, W. E., Gehlbach, S. H., deGruy, F. V., et al. (1988).
   The Duke-UNC Functional Social Support Questionnaire: Measure-
   ment of social support in family practice patients. *Medical Care, 26*(7),
   709-720.
Notes: Probably "state of the art" for family practice research right now.
   The 8-item version is the one currently used by the author.

## MATERNAL SOCIAL SUPPORT INDEX*

Item Number: 21
Item Format: Varied
Key Reference: Pascoe, J. M., Ialongo, N. S., Horn, W. F., et al. (1988). The
   reliability and validity of the Maternal Social Support Index. *Family*
   *Medicine, 20,* 271-276.
Notes: Longer, more specific than the previous three scales. Useful.

## BRIEF ENCOUNTER SOCIAL SUPPORT INSTRUMENT (BESSI)*

Item Number: 3
Item Format: Multiple choice
Key Reference: Frank, S. H., Zyzanski, S. J., & Alemagno, S. *The impact of*
   *stress and support on the medical encounter for upper respiratory infection.*
   Manuscript submitted for publication.
Notes: Includes the Tangible Assistance item from Blake (above). Strong
   results in limited testing.

## SOCIAL AND INSTRUMENTAL ROLE PERFORMANCE

Item Number: 7
Key Reference: Myers, J., Lindenthal, J. J., & Pepper, M. P. (1975). Life
   events, social integration and psychiatric symptomatology. *Journal of*
   *Health and Social Behaviour, 16,* 421-427.

## INDEX OF SOCIAL SUPPORT

Item Number: 13
Key Reference: Gore, S. (1978). The effect of social support in moderating the health consequences of unemployment. *Journal of Health and Social Behaviour, 19*, 157-165.

## SOCIAL SUPPORT SCALE

Item Number: 9
Key Reference: Lin, N., Simenone, R., Ensel, W., & Kuo, W. (1979). Social support, stressful life events and illness: A model and an empirical test. *Journal of Health and Social Behaviour, 20*, 108-119.

## PERSONAL RESOURCE QUESTIONNAIRE (PRQ)

Item Number: Part I-8; Part II-25
Key Reference: Brandt, P. A., & Weinert, C. (1981). The PRQ—A social support measure. *Nursing Research, 30*, 277-280.

## SOCIAL SUPPORT QUESTIONNAIRE

Item Number: Part I-8, Part II-25
Key Reference: Schaefer, C., Coyne, J. C., & Lazarus, R. (1981). The health-related functions of social support. *Journal of Behavioral Medicine, 4*, 381-406.

## SOCIAL SUPPORT INDEX

Item Number: 18
Key Reference: Wilcox, B. L. (1981). Social support, life stress, and psychological adjustment: A test of the buffering hypothesis. *American Journal of Communication Psychology, 9*, 371-386.

## SOCIAL SUPPORT QUESTIONNAIRE

Item Number: 9
Key Reference: Norbeck, J. S., Lindsey, A. M., & Carrieri, V. L. (1981). The development of an instrument to measure social support. *Nursing Research, 30*, 264-269.

## TRADITIONAL SOCIAL SUPPORT INDEX

Item Number: 5

Key Reference: Holahan, C., & Moos, R. (1981). Social support and psychological distress: A longitudinal analysis. *Journal of Abnormal Psychology, 90,* 315-370.

## INDICATORS OF SOCIAL SUPPORT

Item Number: 12
Key Reference: Biegel, E., Naparstek, A. J., & Khan, M. M. (1982). Social support and mental health in urban ethnic neighbourhoods. In E. Biegel & A. J. Naparstek (Eds.), *Community support systems and mental health: Practice, policy, and research.* New York: Springer.

# Broad Spectrum Scales

## CALIFORNIA FAMILY ASSESSMENT SCALES

Subscales: Family structure, family affect, worldview, problem solving, life change, and social network
Key Reference: (Work in progress) Lipkin, M., Fisher, L., Ransom, D., Kokes, R., Phillips, S., & Rudd, P. (1984). *NAPCRG Abstracts.*

## PROFILE OF MOOD STATES (POMS)

Item Number: 65
Item Format: 5-point ordered scale
Subscales: Depression, anxiety, confusion, anger, vigor, fatigue
Key Reference: McNair, D., Lorr, M., & Droppleman, L. (1971). Profile of mood states. San Diego: Educational and Industrial Testing Service.
Notes: Very useful in total or in parts.

## SYMPTOM CHECKLIST-90-R (SCL-90-R)

Item Number: 90
Item Format: 5-point ordered scale
Subscales: Somatization, obsessive/compulsive, interpersonal sensitivity depression, anxiety, hostility, phobic anxiety, paranoid ideation, psychoticism
Key Reference: Derogatis, L. R. (1975). *The SCL-90-R.* Baltimore: Clinical Psychometric Research.
Notes: Very useful in total or in parts.

## GENERAL HEALTH QUESTIONNAIRE (GHQ)

Item Number: 12 to 60 (28-item form suggested)
Subscales: Somatic symptoms, anxiety and insomnia, social dysfunction, and severe depression
Key References: Andrews, G., Tennant, C., Hewson, D. M., & Vaillant, G. E. (1978). Life event stress, social support, coping style, and risk of psychological impairment. *Journal of Nervous Mental Disorders, 166,* 307-316

Morris P. L. P., & Goldberg, R. J. (1989). General health questionnaire. *Psychosomatics, 30,* 290-295. (28-item version)
Notes: Well used. An excellent choice for a short broad-spectrum instrument. Hard to get access without paying for its use.

## MINNESOTA MULTIPHASIC PSYCHIATRIC INVENTORY (MMPI)

Item Number: 566
Item Format: Multiple choice
Key Reference: Hathaway, S. R., & McKinley, J. C. (1940). A multiphasic personality schedule (Minnesota). Part I: Construction of the schedule. *Journal of Psychology, 10,* 249-254.
Notes: The psych standard. Long, need distinct training to interpret the results.

## PSYCHIATRIC EPIDEMIOLOGIC RESEARCH INSTRUMENT (PERI)

Item Number: 149
Item Format: 5-point ordered scale
Subscales: Sadness, despair, anxiety, dread, sexual problems, drinking problems, and 16 more
Key Reference: Social Psychiatry Research Unit. (1977, February). The Psychiatric Epidemiology Research Interview: A report on twenty-two scales, Appendix I to the measurement of psychopathology in the community. New York: Columbia University Press. (mimeographed)

## MILLON BEHAVIORAL HEALTH INVENTORY

Item Number: 150
Item Format: True/False
Subscales: Basic coping styles (introversive, inhibited, cooperative, sociable, confident, forceful, respectful, sensitive), psychogenic attitudes (chronic tension, recent stress, premorbid pessimism, future despair, social alienation, somatic anxiety), psychosomatic correlates (allergic inclination, cardiovascular tendency, gastrointestinal susceptibility),

prognostic indexes (pain treatment responsiveness, life threat reactivity, emotional vulnerability)
Key Reference: Millon, T., Green, C. J., & Meagher, R. B. (1982). *Millon Behavioral Health Inventory*. (Available from National Computer Systems, P.O. Box 1416, Minneapolis, MN 55440)
Notes: Commercially available.

## CORNELL MEDICAL INDEX (CMI)

Item Number: 101
Item Format: Varied
Key Reference: Brodman, K., Erdmann, A. J., Lorge, I., et al. (1949). The Cornell Medical Index: An adjunct to medical interview. *Journal of the American Medical Association, 140*, 530-534.
Notes: Historically important, still in use.

## BRIEF SYMPTOM INVENTORY

Item Number: 52
Item Format: 5-point ordered scale
Subscales: Same as for SCL-90
Key Reference: Derogatis, L. R. (1977). SCL-90-R administration, scoring and procedures manual (Vol. 1). Baltimore: Clinical Psychometric Research.
Notes: The short version of the SCL-90-R. Very useful.

## MIDDLESEX HOSPITAL QUESTIONNAIRE

Item Number: 48
Item Format: Multiple choice
Key Reference: Crown, S., & Crisp, A. H. (1966). A short clinical diagnostic self-rating scale for psychoneurotic patients. *British Journal of Psychiatry, 112*, 917-923.

## MARITAL SATISFACTION INVENTORY

Item Number: 280
Item Format: Varied
Subscales: Affective communication, problem-solving communication, leisure time together, conflict over finances, sexual dissatisfaction, sex role orientation, past family and marital disruption, dissatisfaction with children, conflict over childrearing (also contains a validity scale)
Key Reference: Snyder, D. K. (1979). Multidimensional assessment of marital satisfaction. *Journal of Marriage and the Family, 41*, 121-131.

## DIAGNOSTIC INTERVIEW SCHEDULE (DIS);

Key References: Robins, L. N., Helzer, J., Croughan, J., et. al. (1981). The National Institutes of Mental Health Diagnostic Interview Schedule: Its history, characteristics and validity. *Archives of General Psychiatry, 38,* 381-389.

Katon, W., & Russo, J. (1989). Somatic symptoms and depression. *Journal of Family Practice, 29,* 65-69.

Cadoret, R. J., & Widmer, R. B. (1988). The development of depressive symptoms in the elderly following onset of severe physical illness. *Journal of Family Practice, 27,* 71-76.

Notes: The most important interview-format mental health screen. Adaptation to self-administered format has just begun. Very long but with useful subscales.

## CENTER FOR EPIDEMIOLOGIC STUDIES*

Item Number: 20

Key References: Radloff, L. S. (1977). The CES-D Scale: A self-report depression scale for the use in the general population. *Applied Psychological Measurement, 1,* 385-401.

Pascoe, J. M., Ialongo, N. S., Horn, W. F., et al. (1988). The reliability and validity of the maternal social support index. *Family Medicine, 20,* 271-276.

## MULTIFACTOR HEALTH INVENTORY (MHI)

Item Number: 111

Item Format: 5-point scale

Subscales: Anxiety, depression, hostility, psychosis, obsessive thinking, paranoid thought, impulsivity, and impaired self-esteem

Key References: Hase, H. (1986). *Manual for the Multifactor Health Inventory.* Bismarck, ND: Self-Instruction Press.

Hase, H. D., & Luger, J. A. (1988). Screening for psychosocial problems in primary care. *Journal of Family Practice, 26,* 297-302.

# Family Function

## FAMILY APGAR

Item Number: 5

Item Format: 3- or 5-point ordered scale

Key References: Smilkstein, G., Ashworth, G., & Montano, D. (1982). Validity and reliability of the family APGAR as a test of family function. *Journal of Family Practice, 15,* 303-311.

Reeb, K. G., Graham, A. V., Kitson, G. C., et al. (1986). Defining family in family medicine: Perceived family vs. household structure in an urban black population. *Journal of Family Practice, 23*, 351-355.
Notes: One of the most frequently used tools in family practice despite serious questions about its psychometric characteristics. Very much subject to social desirability bias. Has worked well in a variety of settings despite misgivings. Was especially helpful in an urban black population (see reference above).

## FAMILY FUNCTION INDEX

Item Number: 15
Item Format: Varied
Key Reference: Pless, I. B., & Satterwhite, B. (1973). A measure of family functioning and its application. *Social Science and Medicine, 7*, 613-621.
Notes: The instrument used to validate the Family APGAR. Strongly oriented to traditional nuclear families.

## FAMILY COHESION

Item Number: 8
Item Format: 5-point ordered scale
Key Reference: Speagle, L. E. (1983). *Family cohesion and adaptability.* Unpublished master's thesis, Case Western Reserve University, Cleveland, OH.

## INDEX OF FAMILY RELATIONS

Item Number: 16 or 25
Item Format: 5-point ordered scale
Key References: Hudson, W. (1982). *The clinical measurement package.* Homewood, IL: Dorsey.
    Reeb, K. G., Graham, A. V., Kitson, G. C., et. al. (1986). Defining family in family medicine: Perceived family vs. household structure in an urban black population. *Journal of Family Practice, 23*, 351-355.
Notes: Truncated version used with urban blacks was useful.

## McMASTER FAMILY ASSESSMENT DEVICE (FAD)

Item Number: 53
Item Format: 4 response options
Subscales: Problem solving, communications, roles, affective responsiveness, affective involvement, behavior control

Key Reference: Epstein, N. B., Baldwin, L. M., & Bishop, D. S. (1983). The McMaster family assessment device. *Journal of Marriage and Family Therapy, 9,* 171-180.
Notes: Very nice, somewhat long instrument. Very helpful in teaching about families.

## FACES II; FAMILY ADAPTABILITY AND COHESION SCALES

Item Number: 30
Item Format: 5-point scale
Key References: Olson, D. H., & McCubbin, H. I. (1983). Families: What makes them work. Beverly Hills, CA: Sage.
Clover, R. D., Abell, T., Becker, L. A., et al. (1989). Family functioning and stress as predictors of Influenza B. infection. *Journal of Family Practice, 28,* 535-539.
Notes: Essential for conceptual understanding of families and health. The instrument has become much more practical for use in health settings as it has become shorter. Has worked well in several family practice settings (see reference above). Questions remain regarding how the conceptualization relates to psychometrics, particularly whether the scale can be used in a linear fashion.

## FAMILY ENVIRONMENTAL SCALE

Item Number: 90
Item Format: True/False
Subscales: Family relationship dimension, personal growth dimension, systems maintenance dimension
Key Reference: Moos, R. H. (1974). *The Social Climate Scales: An overview.* Palo Alto, CA: Consulting Psychologists Press.

## FEETHAM FAMILY FUNCTIONING SCALE

Item Number: 21
Key Reference: Roberts, C. S., & Feetham, S. L. (1982). Assessing family functioning across three areas of relationships. *Nursing Research, 31,* 231-235.

## CWRU COMPOSITE FAMILY FUNCTION INSTRUMENT

Item Number: 22 or 31
Item Format: 5-point ordered scale
Key Reference: Reeb, K. G., Graham, A. V., Kitson, G. C., et al. (1986). Defining family in family medicine: Perceived family vs. household

structure in an urban black population. *Journal of Family Practice, 23,* 351-355.
Notes: Mostly validated in urban blacks in this formulation. This is a "cut and paste" instrument using items from the Family APGAR, FACES II, and the Index of Family Relations. Detailed item analysis is available.

## LINDER-PELZ FAMILY FUNCTION QUESTIONNAIRE

Item Number: 9
Item Format: 5-point scale
Key Reference: Linder-Pelz, S., Levy, S., Tamir, A., Spenser, T., & Epstein, L. M. (1984). A measure of family functioning for health care practice and research in Israel. *Journal of Comparative Family Studies, XV*(2), 211-228.

## PERSONAL AUTHORITY IN THE FAMILY SYSTEM QUESTIONNAIRE (PAFS-Q)

Item Number: 84
Item Format: 5-point scale
Subscales: Intergenerational intimacy, intergenerational individuation, personal authority, intergenerational intimidation, intergenerational triangulation, peer intimacy, peer individuation
Key References: Bray, J. H., Williamson, D. S., & Malone, P. E. (1984). Personal authority in the family system: Development of a questionnaire to measure personal authority in intergenerational family processes. *Journal of Marital Family Therapy, 10,* 167-178.
    deGruy, F. V., Dickinson, P., Dickinson, L., et al. (1989). The families of patients with somatization disorder. *Family Medicine, 21,* 438-442.
Notes: Bowenian instrument. Excellent for more detailed study of the family.

## MARITAL AND FAMILY PROBLEMS CHECKLIST

Item Number: 27
Item Format: Yes/No checklist
Key Reference: Geiss, S., & O'Leary, K. (1981). Therapist ratings of frequency and severity of marital problems: Implications for research. *Journal of Marital Family Therapy, 7,* 515-520.
Notes: Checklist format is the only one I am aware of in the literature on family. Goes quickly because of yes/no format.

## DUKE SOCIAL SUPPORT AND STRESS SCALE (DUSOCS)

Item Number: 24
Item Format: 3-point scale
Key Contact: G. Parkerson, Duke University, Department of Family Practice
Notes: Straightforward instrument. Have not seen much data on it yet.

## FAMILY INVENTORY OF LIFE EVENTS (FILE)

Item Number: 71
Item Format: Yes/No
Key Reference: McCubbin, H. I., & Thompson, A. I. (1987). *Family assessment inventories for research and practice*. Madison: University of Wisconsin Press.
Notes: Long, thorough; utility unclear.

## FAMILY SERVICE REQUEST CHECKLIST

Item Number: 15
Item Format: Yes/No checklist
Key Reference: Geiss, S., & O'Leary, K. (1981). Therapist ratings of frequency and severity of marital problems: Implications for research. *Journal of Marital Family Therapy, 7,* 515-520.

## FAMILY ILLNESS BEHAVIOR SCALE

Item Number: 27
Item Format: 5-point scale
Key Contact: P. Dickinson, University of South Alabama, Department of Family Medicine

# Marital Satisfaction

## DYADIC INTERACTION SCALE

Item Number: 32
Item Format: Varied
Key Reference: Spanier, G. B. (1976). Measuring dyadic adjustment: New scales for assessing the quality of marriage and similar dyads. *Journal of Marriage and the Family, 38,* 15-28.
Notes: Well used, fairly flexible for nontraditional relationships.

## SHORT MARITAL ADJUSTMENT TEST

Item Number: 15
Item Format: 6-point ordered scale
Key Reference: Locke, H. J., & Wallace, K. M. (1959, August). Short marital adjustment and prediction tests: Their reliability and validity. *Marriage and Family Living, 21*(3), 251-255.
Notes: One of the most commonly used marital assessments. Fits best in traditional marital settings.

## AREAS OF CHANGE QUESTIONNAIRE

Item Format: 7-point scale
Key Reference: Margolin, G., Talovic, S., & Weinstein, C. (in press). The areas of change questionnaire: A practical approach to marital assessment. *Journal of Consulting and Clinical Psychology.*

## SHORT RELATIONSHIP INVENTORY

Item Number: 15
Item Format: 5-point ordered scale
Key Reference: Schumm, W. R., Jurich, A. P., & Bollman, S. R. (1980). The dimensionality of an abbreviated Relationship Inventory for couples. *Journal of Psychology, 105,* 225-230.

## CONFLICT TACTICS SCALE

Item Number: 19
Item Format: Frequency count
Key Reference: Straus, M. A. (1979). Measuring intrafamily conflict and violence: The conflict tactics (CT) scales. *Journal of Marriage and the Family, 41,* 75-88.

## RYLE MARITAL PATTERNS TEST

Item Number: 38
Item Format: Varied
Subscales: Affection given, affection received, domination
Key Reference: Heins, T. J., & Yelland, J. H. (1981). Validity studies on the Ryle Marital Patterns Test. *British Journal of Medical Psychology, 54,* 51-58.

## MARITAL SATISFACTION QUESTIONNAIRE

Item Number: 36
Item Format: Variable
Key Reference: Madden, M. E., & Janoff-Bulman, R. (1981). Blame, control, and marital conflict: Wives' attributions for conflict in marriage. *Journal of Marriage and the Family, 43,* 663-674.

## AREAS OF CHANGE QUESTIONNAIRE

Item Number: 34
Key Reference: Weiss, R. L., Hops, H., & Patterson, G. R. (1973). A framework for conceptualizing marital conflict. In L. A. Hamerlynck, L. C. Hardy, & E. J. Marsh (Eds.), *Behavior change: Methodology, concepts, and practices.* Champaign, IL: Research Press.

## BRODERICK COMMITMENT SCALE

Item Number: 1
Item Format: 1-paragraph definition that the subject rates on scale 1 to 100
Key Reference: Broderick, J. E. (1981). A method for derivation of areas for assessment in marital relationships. *American Journal of Family Therapy, 9,* 25-34.

## MARITAL SATISFACTION SCALE

Item Number: 48
Item Format: 5-point scale
Key Reference: Roach, A. J., Frazier, L. P., & Bowden, S. R. (1981, August). The Marital Satisfaction Scale: Development of a measure for intervention research. *Journal of Marriage and the Family, ,* 537-546.

## RELATIONSHIP BELIEF INVENTORY

Item Number: Three 12-item scales
Subscales: Disagreement is destructive, mind reading is expected, partners cannot change
Key Reference: Eidelson, R. J., & Epstein, N. (1982). Cognition and relationship maladjustment: Development of a measure of dysfunctional relationship beliefs. *Journal of Consulting and Clinical Psychology, 50,* 715-720.
Notes: Wonderful instrument to use as an adjunct in brief marital counseling.

# Communication

## PRIMARY COMMUNICATION INVENTORY

Item Number: 25
Key Reference: Locke, H. J., Sabagh, G., & Thomas, M. (1956). Correlates of primary communication and empathy. *Research Studies of the State College of Washington, 24,* 116-124.

## VERBAL PROBLEM CHECKLIST

Item Number: 27
Item Format: 5-point ordered scale
Key Reference: Chavez, R. E., Samuel, V., & Haynes, S. N. (1981, November). *Validity of the Verbal Problems Checklist.* Paper presented at the annual meeting of the Association for Advancement of Behaviour Therapy, Toronto.

## MARITAL COMMUNICATIONS INVENTORY

Item Number: 19 or 46
Key Reference: Schumm, W. R., Race, G. S., Morris, J. E., Anderson, S. A., Griffin, C. L., McCutchen, M. B., & Benigas, J. E. (1981). Dimensionality of the marital communication inventory and marital conventionalization: A third report. *Psychological Reports, 48,* 163-171.

# Health Risk Behaviors

## HEALTH PRACTICES

Item Number: 7
Item Format: Yes/No
Subscales: Exercise, alcohol, smoking, nutrition
Key Reference: Belloc, N., & Breslow, L. (1972). Relationship of physical health status and health practices. *Preventive Medicine, 1,* 409-421.
Notes: Nice short companion piece to consider including in studies even when it is not the focus.

# Alcoholism

## MICHIGAN ALCOHOL SCREENING TEST (MAST)

Item Number: 25
Item Format: Yes/No
Key Reference: Selzer, M. L. (1971). The Michigan Alcoholism Screening
Instrument (MAST). *American Journal of Psychiatry, 127,* 1653.
Notes: The "gold standard" for pencil-and-paper diagnosis of alcoholism.
Still among the most useful instruments available for teaching, patient
care, and research.

## SHORT MICHIGAN ALCOHOL SCREENING TEST (SMAST)

Item Format: Yes/No
Key Reference: Selzer, M., Vinokur, A., & Van Rooijen, L. (1975). A self-
administered Short Michigan Alcoholism Screening Test (SMAST).
*Journal of Studies on Alcohol, 36,* 117.

## CAGE

Item Number: 4
Item Format: Yes/No
Key Reference: Mayfield, D., McLeod, G., & Hall, P. (1974). The CAGE
Questionnaire: Validation of a new alcoholism screening instrument.
*American Journal of Psychiatry, 131,* 1121-1123.
Notes: Important conceptually. Excellent for teaching. Good for inclusion
as brief alcohol assessment.

## SEVERITY OF ALCOHOL DEPENDENCE

Item Number: 33
Item Format: Yes/No
Key Reference: Stockwell, T., Hodgson, R., Edwards, G., Taylor, C., &
Rankin, H. (1979). The development of a questionnaire to measure
severity of alcohol dependence, *British Journal of Addiction, 74,* 79-87.

## MUNICH ALCOHOLISM TEST

Item Number: 24 (patient), 7 (physician)
Item Format: Yes/No

Key Reference: Feuerlein, W., et al. (1980). Diagnosis of Alcoholism: The Munich Alcohol Screening Test (MALT). In M. Galantes (Ed.), *Currents in alcoholism* (Vol. III) (pp. 137-147).

## SELF-ADMINISTERED ALCOHOL SCREENING TEST

Item Number: 34
Item Format: Yes/No
Key Reference: Swenson, W., & Morse, R. M. (1975). Use of the Self-Administered Alcoholism Screening Test (SAAST) in a medical center. *Mayo Clinic Proceedings, 50,* 204-208.

# Tobacco Dependence

## FAGERSTROM TOLERANCE QUESTIONNAIRE

Item Number: 8
Item Format: Varied
Key Reference: Fagerstrom K. O. (1978). Measuring the degree of physical dependence to tobacco smoking with reference to individualization of treatment. *Addictive Behaviours, 3,* 235-241.
Notes: First and best measure of level of tobacco dependence.

## THE SMOKER'S CAGE

Item Number: 4
Item Format: Yes/No
Key Contact: S. Frank, Department of Family Medicine, Case Western Reserve University, Cleveland, OH. Publication pending.
Notes: Excellent clinical tool for taking a tobacco use history.

# Eating Disorders

## BULIMIA TEST (BULIT)

Item Number: 32
Item Format: Multiple choice
Key Reference: Smith, M. C., & Thelen, M. N. (1984). Development and validation of a test for bulimia. *Journal of Consulting and Clinical Psychology, 52,* 863-872.
Notes: DSM-III-based instrument.

## COMPULSIVE EATING SCALE (CES)

Item Number: 8
Item Format: Multiple choice
Key Reference: Kagan, D. M., & Squires, R. L. (1984). *Eating disorders among adolescents: Patterns and prevalence. Adolescence, 19,* 15-29.
Notes: Developed for use with adolescents but has potential for use in adults too. Short and usable.

## Somatization

### DIAGNOSTIC INTERVIEW SCHEDULE (DIS); SOMATIZATION SUBSCALE*

Key References: Robins, L. N., Helzer, J., Croughan, J., et al. (1981). The National Institutes of Mental Health Diagnostic Interview Schedule: Its history, characteristics and validity. *Archives of General Psychiatry, 38,* 381-389.
Katon, W., & Russo, J. (1989). Somatic symptoms and depression. *Journal of Family Practice, 29,* 65-69.
Cadoret, R. J., & Widmer, R. B. (1988). The development of depressive symptoms in the elderly following onset of severe physical illness. *Journal of Family Practice, 27,* 71-76.
Notes: Useful subscale of the DIS.

### SYMPTOM CHECKLIST-90-R (SCL-90-R)

Item Number: 9
Item Format: 5-point ordered scale
Key Reference: Derogatis, L. R. (1975). *The SCL-90-R.* Baltimore: Clinical Psychometric Research.
Notes: The somatization scale of the SCL-90-R is particularly useful.

### SOMATIZATION SCREEN

Item Number: 7
Item Format: Interview
Key Reference: deGruy, F. V., Columbia, L., & Dickinson, P. (1987). Somatization disorder in a family practice. *Journal of Family Practice, 25,* 45-51.

# Reason for Visit

## PATIENT REQUESTS*

Key Reference: Like, R. C. (1984). *Patient requests in family practice: A negotiated approach to clinical care.* Unpublished master's thesis, Case Western Reserve University, Cleveland, OH.

# Coping

## SENSE OF MASTERY*

Item Number: 7
Key Reference: Pearlin, L. I., and Schooler, C. (1978). The structure of coping. *Journal of Health and Social Behaviour, 19,* 2-21.
Notes: Probably most commonly used in primary care. Also used as a "locus of control" instrument.

## COPING RESPONSE*

Item Number: 19
Item Format: Asks coping response to last stressful experience.
Key References: Billings, A. G., & Moos, R. H. (1981). The role of coping response and social resources in attenuating the stress of life events. *Journal of Behavioral Medicine, 4,* 139-157.
Blake, R. L., & Vandiver, T. A. (1988). The association of health with stressful life changes, social supports and coping. *Family Practice Research Journal, 7,* 205-218.

## LOEVINGER SENTENCE COMPLETION TEST

Key Reference: Loevinger, J. (1979). Construct validity of the Sentence Completion Test of Ego Development. *Applied Psychological Measurement, 3,* 281-211.

## DEFENSE MECHANISM INVENTORY

Item Number: 20
Item Format: 7-point ordered scale
Subscales: Turning against self, turning against object, projection, principalization, reversal

Key Reference: Gleser, G. C., & Ihilevich, D. (1969). An objective instrument for measuring defense mechanisms. *Journal of Consulting and Clinical Psychology, 33,* 51-60.

## BEHAVIORAL ATTRIBUTES OF PSYCHOSOCIAL COMPETENCE

Item Number: 45
Item Format: Forced choice
Key Reference: Tyler, F. B. (1978). Individual psychological competence: A personality configuration. *Educational and Psychological Measurement, 38,* 309-323.

## MEANS-ENDS PROBLEM-SOLVING PROCEDURE

Item Number: 10 scenarios
Item Format: Open-ended
Key Reference: Platt, J. J., & Spivack, G. (1975). *Manual for the Means-Ends Problem-Solving Procedure (MEPS): A measure of interpersonal cognitive problem-solving skill.* Philadelphia: Hahnemann Medical College and Hospital, Hahnemann Community Mental Health/Mental Retardation Center.

## EMOTIONAL MEANS-ENDS PROBLEM-SOLVING PROCEDURE

Item Number: 10 scenarios
Item Format: Open-ended
Key Reference: Platt, J. J., & Spivack, G. (1977). *Measures of interpersonal problem-solving for adults and adolescents.* Philadelphia: Hahnemann Medical College and Hospital, Hahnemann Community Mental Health/Mental Retardation Center.

## JOFFE AND NADITCH COPING SCALES

Item Number: 31 to 36 per subscale
Item Format: True/False
Subscales: Isolation, intellectualization, rationalization, denial, projection, regression, displacement, reaction formation, repression, doubt
Key Reference: Joffe, P. E., & Naditch, M. (1977). Paper and pencil measures of coping and defense processes. In N. Haan (Ed.), *Coping and defending: Processes of self-environment organization.* New York: Academic.

## WAYS OF COPING

Item Number: 68
Item Format: Yes/No
Key Reference: Folkman, S., & Lazarus, R. S. (1980). An analysis of coping in a middle-aged community sample. *Journal of Health and Social Behaviour, 21,* 219-239.

## COPING OPERATIONS PREFERENCE

Item Number: 30
Item Format: 6 brief stories with 5 responses each on a 7-point ordered scale
Subscales: Denial, isolation, projection, regression, turning against self
Key Reference: Schultz, W. C. (1967). *The FIRO Scales manual.* Palo Alto, CA: Consulting Psychologists Press.

# Self-Image/Esteem

## ROSENBERG SELF-ESTEEM SCALE*

Item Number: 10
Item Format: 4-point scale
Key References: Rosenberg, M. (1965). *Society and the adolescent self-image.* Princeton, NJ: Princeton University Press.
Antonucci, T. C., Peggs, J. F., & Marquez, J. T. (1989). The relationship between self-esteem and physical health in a family practice population. *Family Practice Research Journal, 9,* 65-72.

## SELF-CONCEPT SEMANTIC DIFFERENTIAL SCALE

Item Number: 12
Item Format: Semantic differential, 7-point scale
Key Reference: Avillo, L. J. (1971). *The effectiveness of a teaching approach on self-concept in post-myocardial infarction patients.* Unpublished master's thesis, University of Arizona, Tucson.

## INDEX OF SELF-ESTEEM (HUDSON 9)

Item Number: 25
Item Format: 5-point ordered scale
Key Reference: Hudson, W. (1982). *The clinical measurement package.* Homewood, IL: Dorsey.

## PEARLIN SELF-ESTEEM

Item Number: 10
Item Format: 5-point ordered scale
Key Reference: Pearlin, L. I., & Schooler, C. (1978). The structure of coping. *Journal of Health and Social Behaviour, 19,* 2-21.

## FEELINGS OF INADEQUACY SCALE

Item Number: 20
Item Format: 5-point ordered scale
Key Reference: Eagly, A. H. (1967). Involvement as a determinant of response to favourable and unfavourable information. *Journal of Personality and Social Psychology, 7*(3), 1-15. (monograph)

## SELF-ESTEEM INVENTORY

Item Number: 25
Item Format: 2 choice responses
Key Reference: Coopersmith, S. (1967). *The antecedents of self-esteem.* San Francisco: Freeman.

## SHERWOOD SELF-CONCEPT INVENTORY

Item Number: 15
Item Format: 11-point graphic bipolar scale
Key Reference: Sherwood, J. J. (1970). Self-actualization and self-identity theory. *Personality, 1,* 41-63.

# Personality

## JENKINS ACTIVITY SURVEY

Key Reference: Jenkins, C. D., Zyzanski, S. J., & Rosenman, R. H. (1976). Risk of new myocardial infarction in middle-aged men with manifest coronary heart disease. *Circulation, 53,* 342-347.

## SHORT TYPE A SCALE*

Item Number: 6-item weighted scale
Item Format: Forced choice

Key Reference: Flynn, S. P., & Zyzanski, S. J. (1987). Type A behaviour in married couples in a family practice population. *Family Medicine, 19,* 433-437.
Notes: Short, reliable, useful.

## MYERS-BRIGGS TYPE INDICATOR

Item Number: 126
Item Format: Forced choice
Key Reference: Myers, I. (1962). *Manual: The Myers-Briggs Type Indicator.* Palo Alto, CA: Consulting Psychologists Press.
Notes: Well researched and used in medical schools and family medicine education. Excellent "process" instrument for use in group or team development.

## KEIRSEY TEMPERAMENT SORTER

Item Number: 70
Item Format: Forced choice
Key Reference: Keirsey, D., & Bates, M. (1978). *Please understand me: Character and temperament types.* Del Mar, CA: Prometheus Nemesis.

## TAYLOR JOHNSON TEMPERAMENT ANALYSIS*

Subscales: Personality traits
Key References: Taylor, R. M., & Morrison, W. L. (1980). *Taylor Johnson Temperament Analysis handbook.* Los Angeles: Psychological Publications.
Parker, J., & Rodney, W. (1986). Temperament and stress factors predictive of choosing to leave after one year of residency. *Family Medicine, 18,* 308-310.

# Functional Status/Patient Perception of Health and Illness

## DUKE-UNC HEALTH PROFILE (DUHP)*

Item Number: 63
Item Format: 3-point scale
Subscales: Symptoms, physical function, social function, emotional function
Key References: Parkerson, G. R., Gehlbach, S. H., Wagner, E. H., et al. (1981). The Duke-UNC Health Profile: An adult health status measure for primary care. *Medical Care, 19,* 806-823.

Blake, R. L. Vandiver, T. A., Zweig, S. C., et al. (1986). Evaluation of health status measure in adults with high psychosocial risk. *Family Practice Research Journal, 5,* 158-166.
Notes: An important instrument for primary care. Very useful as an outcome measure or an independent variable. The mini version is more practical in a clinical setting.

## MINI DUKE-UNC HEALTH PROFILE (MINI DUHP)*

Item Number: 10
Item Format: 3-point scale
Subscales: Symptoms, physical function, social function, emotional function
Key Reference: Blake, R. L., & Vandiver, T. A. (1986). The reliability and validity of a 10-item measure of functional status. *Journal of Family Practice, 23*(5), 455-459.
Notes: Widely used, well tested, extremely "functional" measure of functional status.

## OLDER AMERICANS RESOURCES AND SERVICES QUESTIONNAIRE (OARS)*

Item Number: 101
Item Format: Interview-administered 6-point scale
Subscales: Assesses the status of five areas of function: social, economic, physical health, mental health, self-care capacity
Key References: Fillenbaum, G. G., & Symer, M. (1981). The development, validity and reliability of OARS multidimensional functional assessment questionnaire. *Journal of Gerontology, 36,* 428-434.
Zyzanski, S. J., Medalie, J. H, Ford, A. B., et al. (1989). Living arrangements and well-being of the elderly. *Family Medicine, 21,* 199-205.

## RAND HEALTH STATUS SCALE (COOP VERSION)*

Item Number: 23
Item Format: Multiple choice
Subscales: Assesses the status of seven areas of function: self-care limitations (1 item), mobility limitations (3 items), physical ability (4 items), role activity limitation (3 items), anxiety (5 items), depression (3), validity (4)
Key Reference: Nelson, E. C., Conger, B., Douglas, R., et al. (1983). Functional health status levels of primary care patients. *Journal of the American Medical Association, 249,* 3331-3338.

## NATIONAL HEALTH SURVEY MONTHLY MORBIDITY*

Subscales: Hospital days, bed days, missed work/school days, reduced activity for health problem days, and number of physician visits
Key References: National Center for Health Statistics. (1978). *Disability Days: US, 1975.* (DHEW Pub. No., 78-1546). Washington, DC: Government Printing Office.
Blake R. L., Vandiver, T. A., Zweig, S. C., et al. (1986). Evaluation of health status measure in adults with high psychosocial risk. *Family Practice Research Journal, 5,* 158-166.
Notes: "Gold standard" against which most tests of functional status were originally measured. Shorter, validated instruments can now often take its place.

## HEALTH ILLNESS QUESTIONNAIRE

Item Number: 8
Item Format: Forced choice, 4 options
Key Reference: Boire, M. I. (1976). *A study of the relationship between trait-powerlessness and situational powerlessness in the hospitalized patient.* Unpublished master's thesis, University of California, Los Angeles.

## SICK ROLE ACCEPTANCE

Item Number: 20
Item Format: Semantic differential, 7-point scale
Key Reference: Brown, J. S., & Rawlinson, M. E. (1975). Relinquishing the sick role following open-heart surgery. *Journal of Health and Social Behaviour, 16,* 12-27.

## HEALTH SELF-CONCEPT

Item Number: 7
Item Format: Yes/No
Key Reference: Jacox, A., & Stewart, M. (1973). *Psychosocial contingencies of the pain experience.* (DHEW Grant No. NU-00387-02). Iowa City: University of Iowa.

## HEALTH OPINION SURVEY

Key Reference: MacMillan, A. M. (1957). The Health Opinion Survey: Technique for estimating prevalence of psychoneurotic and related types of disorder in communities [Monograph]. *Psychological Reports, 3*(Suppl. 7), 325-339.

## IRRATIONAL BELIEFS TEST

Item Format: 3 scales
Key Reference: Jones, R. G. (1968). *A factored measure of Ellis' Irrational Belief System with personality and maladjustment correlates.* Unpublished doctoral dissertation, Texas Technological College.

## SICKNESS IMPACT PROFILE

Item Number: 146 or 235
Item Format: Varied
Key Reference: Pollard, W. E., Bobbitt, R. A., Bergner, M., Martin, D. P., & Gilson, B. S. (1976). The Sickness Impact Profile: Reliability of a health status measure. *Medical Care, 14*(2), 146-155.
Notes: Often-used instrument. Long.

## Wellness

## GENERALIZED CONTENTMENT SCALE

Item Number: 25
Item Format: 5-point ordered scale
Key Reference: Hudson, W. (1982). *The clinical measurement package.* Homewood, IL; Dorsey.

## RAND INDEX OF VALIDITY*

Item Number: 4
Item Format: Multiple choice
Key Reference: Brook, R. H., Ware, J. E., Jr., Davies-Avery, A., et al. (1979). Overview of adult health status measures fielded in Rand's Health Insurance study. *Medical Care, 17*(suppl), 1-55.

## GENERAL WELL-BEING SCHEDULE

Item Number: 18
Item Format: 14 items with 6 response categories, 4 items with 11
Key Reference: Dupuy, H. J. (1973). *Developmental rationale, substantive, derivative, and conceptual relevance of general well-being* Washington, DC: National Center for Health Statistics. (draft working paper)

# Pain

## PAIN AND DISTRESS SCALE

Item Number: 20
Item Format: 4-point ordered scale
Key Reference: Zung, W. K. (1983). A self-rating pain and distress scale. *Psychosomatics, 24*(10), 887-894.

## PAIN DESCRIPTION INDEX

Item Number: 10
Item Format: Forced choice, 4 responses
Key Reference: Rasmussen, S. R. (1974). *Chronic pain: Relationship of personality variables and pain description.* Unpublished master's thesis, University of Illinois, Urbana.

## ACUTE PAIN ASSESSMENT AND MANAGEMENT*

Item Format: 10-point scale
Key Reference: Sutherland, J. E., Wesley, R. M., Cole, P. M., Nesvacil, L. J., Daly, M. L., & Gepner, G. J. (1988). Differences and similarities between patient and physician perceptions of pain. *Family Medicine, 20,* 343-346.

## PATIENT PAST PAIN EXPERIENCE INTERVIEW

Item Number: 14
Item Format: Open-ended
Key Reference: Jacox, A., & Stewart, M. (1973). Psychosocial contingencies of the pain experience (DHEW Grant No. NU-00387-02). Iowa City: University of Iowa.

# Locus of Control

## HEALTH LOCUS OF CONTROL*

Item Number: 11
Item Format: 6-point ordered scale
Key References: Wallston, B. S., Wallston, K. A., Gordon, D., & Maides, S. A. (1976). Development and validation of the health locus of control (HLC) scale. *Journal of Consulting and Clinical Psychology, 44*(4), 580-585.

Zweig, S., LeFevre, M., & Kruse, J. (1988). The health belief model and attendance for prenatal care. *Family Practice Research Journal, 8,* 32-41.

## Patient Satisfaction

### PATIENT SATISFACTION QUESTIONNAIRE*

Item Number: 18 or 43
Item Format: 5-point scale
Subscales: Access to care, availability, continuity, humaneness, quality/
competence, general
Key References: Ware, J. E., & Snyder, M. K. (1975). Dimensions of patient
attitude regarding doctors and medical care services. *Medical Care, 13,*
669.

Cherkdin, D. C., Hart, G., & Rosenblatt, R. A. (1988). Patient satisfaction with family physicians and general internists: Is there a difference? *Journal of Family Practice, 26,* 543-551. (18-item scale)

Rodney, W., Quigley, C. B., Werblun, M. N., et al. (1986). Satisfaction of continuity patients in a family medicine residency: Validation of a measurement tool. *Family Practice Research Journal, 5,* 167-176.

Notes: Probably the most commonly used satisfaction instrument. A notoriously difficult outcome to demonstrate differences with.

### PATIENT SATISFACTION WITH HEALTH CARE

Item Number: 21
Item Format: Multiple choice
Key Reference: Linn, L. (1975, Fall). Factors associated with patient evaluation of health care. *Health and Society, 53*(4), 531-548.

### SATISFACTION WITH MEDICAL CARE

Item Number: 41
Item Format: 9-point scale
Key Reference: Zyzanski, S. J., Hulka, B. S., & Cassel, J. C. (1974). Scale for the measurement of "Satisfaction" with medical care: Modifications in content, format and scoring. *Medical Care, 12*(7), 611-620.

## Humanism

### PATIENT PERCEPTION OF PHYSICIAN HUMANISM*

Item Number: 24

Item Format: Graphic scales
Key Reference: Hauck, F.R., Zyzanski, S. J., Alemagno, S. A., Medalie, J. H. (1990). Patient perceptions of Humanism in physicians: Effects on positive health behaviors. *Family Medicine, 22*(6), 447-452.

## Sexual Function

### SEXUAL FUNCTION QUESTIONNAIRE*

Item Number: 7 to 12 items for each of 15 different sexual problems
Item Format: Multiple choice
Subscales: Sexual desire, arousal, orgasm, gender identity, sexual orientation, sexual intention, dyspareunia, emotional dissatisfaction, inability to relax
Key Reference: Schein, M., Zyzanski, S. J., Levine, S., et al. (1988). The frequency of sexual problems among family practice patients. *Family Practice Research Journal, 7*(3), 122-134.

### SURVEY OF SEXUAL PROBLEMS CARE (SSPC)*

Item Number: 66
Key Reference: Nease, D. E., & Liese, B. S. (1987). Perception and treatment of sexual problems. *Family Medicine, 19*, 468-470.

### SEX PROBLEMS IN FAMILY PRACTICE QUESTIONNAIRE*

Item Number: 102
Key Reference: Houge, D. R. (1988). Sex problems in family practice. *Family Practice Research Journal, 7*(3), 135-140.

### INDEX OF SEXUAL SATISFACTION

Item Number: 25
Item Format: 5-point ordered scale
Key Reference: Hudson, W. (1982). *The clinical measurement package.* Homewood, IL; Dorsey.

### SEXUAL AROUSAL INVENTORY

Item Number: 28

Key Reference: Hoon, E. F., Hoon, P., & Wincze, J. (1976). An inventory for the measurement of female sexual arousability. *Archives of Sexual Behavior, 5*, 291-300.

## SEXUAL INTERACTION SURVEY

Key Reference: LoPiccolo, J., & Steger, J. C. (1974). The Sexual Interaction Inventory: A new instrument for assessment of sexual dysfunction. *Archives of Sexual Behaviour, 3*, 585-595.

## Anomy

### ANOMY

Item Number: 9
Item Format: Agree/Disagree
Key Reference: McCloskey, H., & Scharr, J. (1965). Psychological dimensions of anomy. *American Social Review, 30*(1), 14-40.

### ANOMIA

Item Number: 5 or 9
Item Format: Agree/Disagree
Key Reference: Srole, L. (1956). Social integration and certain corollaries. *American Social Review, 21*, 709-716.

### ALIENATION VIA REJECTION

Item Number: 18
Item Format: 6-point ordered scale
Key Reference: Robinson, J., & Shaver, P. (1973). *Measures of social psychological attitudes*. Ann Arbor, MI: Institute for Social Research.

## Pediatric Psychosocial Tests

### CHILD HEALTH QUESTIONNAIRE

Item Number: 20
Item Format: 3-point ordered scale
Key Reference: Butler, A. C. (1975). The child health questionnaire: Preliminary data. *Psychology in the Schools, 12*, 153-160.

## PAEDIATRIC BEHAVIORAL QUESTIONNAIRE

Item Number: 28
Item Format: Yes/No
Key Reference: Tasem, W. M., Dasteel, J. C., & Goldenberg, E. D. (1974). Psychiatric screening and brief intervention in a paediatric program utilizing allied health personnel. *Journal of Orthopsychiatry, 44*(4), 568-578.

## WASHINGTON SYMPTOM CHECKLIST

Item Number: 67
Item Format: 4-point ordered scale
Key Reference: Wimberger, H. C., & Gregory, R. J. (1968). A behavior checklist for use in child psychiatry clinics. *Journal of the American Academy of Child Psychiatry, 7,* 677-688.

## HOME OBSERVATION FOR THE MEASUREMENT OF THE ENVIRONMENT (HOME)

Item Number: 45
Item Format: Yes/No
Key Reference: Caldwell, B. M. (1967). Descriptive evaluations of child development and of developmental settings. *Paediatrics, 40,* 46-54.

## INFANT TEMPERAMENT QUESTIONNAIRE

Key Reference: Bradley-Johnson, S., King, L. W., King, D. W., et al. (1985). The infant temperament questionnaire as a screening measure to aid the family physician: A pilot study. *Family Practice Research Journal, 5,* 93-98.

## Geriatric Psychosocial Tests

## OLDER AMERICANS RESOURCES AND SERVICES QUESTIONNAIRE (OARS)*

Item Number: 101
Item Format: Interview-administered 6-point scale
Subscales: Assesses the status of five areas of function: social, economic physical health, mental health, and self-care capacity
Key References: Fillenbaum, G. G., & Symer, M. (1981). The development validity and reliability of the OARS multidimensional functional assessment questionnaire. *Journal of Gerontology, 36,* 428-434.

Zyzanski, S.., Medalie, J. H., Ford, A. B., et al. (1989). Living arrangements and well-being of the elderly. *Family Medicine, 21*, 199-205.

## INDEX OF ADL

Item Number: 6
Item Format: Observational, multiple choice
Key Reference: Katz, S., & Akpom, A. (1976). A measure of primary sociobiologic functions. *International Journal of Health Services, 6*, 493-508.

## THE STOKES-GORDON STRESS SCALE (SGSS)

Item Number: 104
Item Format: Checklist
Key Reference: Stokes, S. A., & Gordon, S. E. (1988). Development of an instrument to measure stress in the older adult. *Nursing Research, 37*(1), 16-18.

## PSYCHOSOCIAL FUNCTION SCALE

Item Number: 8
Item Format: Fully anchored 5-point scale
Key Reference: Putnam, P. A. (1973). Nurse awareness and psychosocial function in the aged. *The Gerontologist, 13*(2), 163-166.

## GERIATRIC SOCIAL READJUSTMENT RATING SCALE

Item Number: 35
Key Reference: Amster, L. E., & Krauss, H. H. (1974). The relationship between life crisis and mental deterioration in old age. *International Jounal of Aging and Human Development, 5*, 51-55.

# Mental Status

## SHORT PORTABLE MENTAL STATUS QUESTIONNAIRE

Item Number: 10
Item Format: Short answers
Key Reference: Pfeiffer, E. (1975). A short portable mental status questionnaire for the assessment of organic brain deficit in elderly patients. *American Geriatrics Society, 23*, 433.
Notes: Highly useful in research and practice.

## MENTAL STATUS INDEX

Item Number: 20
Item Format: Varied
Key Reference: Gurin, G., Veroff, J., & Feld, S. (1960). *Americans view their mental health.* New York: Basic Books.

## ORIENTATION-MEMORY-CONCENTRATION TEST

Item Number: 6
Item Format: Short answers
Key Reference: Katzman, R. (1983). Orientation-Memory-Concentration Test. *American Journal of Psychiatry, 140,* 734.

## MINI MENTAL STATUS TEST

Item Number: 11
Item Format: Varied
Key Reference: Folstein, M. F., Folstein, S. E., & McHugh, P. R. (1975). Mini-mental state: A practical method for grading the cognitive state of patients for the clinician. *Journal of Psychiatric Research, 12,* 189-198.
Notes: Highly useful in research and practice.

# Name Index

# Subject Index

# About the Authors

**Martin J. Bass,** MD, MSc, FCFP, is Professor of Family Medicine and Epidemiology at The University of Western Ontario. He is the Director of the Centre for Studies in Family Medicine and conducts research on preventive care, appropriate technology for family practice, and quality of care. He has a special interest in refining research methods for the family practice setting.

**David W. Beaufait,** MD, is in full-time community practice of Family Medicine. Major research interests include the management of common clinical problems in community practice. Prior work involved the primary care management of headache with the Ambulatory Sentinel Practice Network (ASPN) and influenza surveillance with the ASPN-CDC-AAFP Influenza Surveillance Network. Recent research has focused on the primary care management and functional health status of patients with Type II diabetes in community practice, with the Dartmouth COOP Project and ASPN. Results have been reported in MMWR and in NAFCRG and AAFP forums. Publications and presentation of recent studies are in preparation.

**Cindy I. Carlson,** Ph.D., an Associate Professor and licensed psychologist in the Department of Educational Psychology at the University of Texas at Austin, is a recognized scholar in the area of family assessment. She is coauthor with H. D. Grotevant of the book *Family Assessment: A Guide for Clinicians and Researchers* and has published on family assessment issues in books and such journals as the *Journal of Family Psychology*. Her research interests also include family systems therapy as evidenced by her most recent book *Handbook of Family-School Intervention: A Systems*

*Approach,* coedited with M. J. Fine. She received her Ph.D. from Indiana University.

**Benjamin F. Crabtree,** Ph.D., Medical Anthropologist and Assistant Professor in the Department of Family Medicine at the University of Connecticut, is cofounder of the Qualitative Research Interest Group within the North American Primary Care Research Group and has published in books and such journals as the *Journal of Clinical Epidemiology, Medical Care,* and *Family Medicine.* He and William Miller are co-editors of the volume on *Doing Qualitative Research in Primary Care: Multiple Strategies* (in press).

**Larry Culpepper,** MD, MPH, is Research Director at the Memorial Hospital of Rhode Island/Brown University Department of Family Medicine. He is President of the North American Primary Care Research Group and helps direct the International Primary Care Network. He has made frequent contributions to the development of Family Medicine Research over the past 15 years, including publications in the *Journal of the American Medical Association, British Medical Journal, Journal of Family Medicine,* and *Family Practice.*

**Earl V. Dunn,** MD, FCFP(C), was born in the Province of Quebec in 1931, educated in Quebec and New Brunswick, and graduated form Mc Gill University Medical School in 1960. He did a 2-year General Practice residency in Kansas City, Missouri, and then entered practice in a mining community in the Province of Quebec. After 5 years, in 1968, he became a full-time member of the Faculty of Medicine, University of Toronto. In 1982 he became a Professor in the Department of Family and Community Medicine. He is also a Professor in the Centre for Studies in Medical Education, University of Toronto. He has specific interests in medical decision making, telemedicine, and resource utilization and the economics of health care delivery and has published in all these fields.

**Lorraine E. Ferris,** Ph.D., is Assistant Professor in the Department of Behaviourial Science, Faculty of Medicine at the University of Toronto and a Research Associate in the Clinical Epidemiology Unit at Sunnybrook Health Science Centre, Toronto, Ontario. She is currently Chair, Section on Community Psychology for the Canadian Psychological Association and is actively involved in community health research. Her research interests include such areas as instrument development for primary care and quality-of-life studies, components of service delivery, and program evaluation.

**Scott H. Frank,** MD, is Residency Director and Assistant Professor in the Department of Family Medicine at Case Western Reserve University School of Medicine. His interest in documentation of the impact of psychosocial problems on health behavior in physical health have led to extensive work in measurement of psychosocial variables. His special interests include clinical assessment of individual and family stress. His work has been published in books and such journals as the *Journal of Family Practice* and *Primary Care*. He received his MD from the University of Michigan and a Master of Science in Family Medicine from Case Western Reserve University.

**Edmee Franssen,** BSc, MSc, is a Biostatistitian and Research Associate with the Department of Family and Community Medicine, Sunnybrook Health Science Centre, University of Toronto. As a member of the Primary Care Research Unit, she is involved in the planning and organization of all phases of its research activities; as well, she is a consultant in statistical and methodological issues for the unit and for the residents.

**Curtis G. Hames,** MD., is a Clinical Professor, Department of Epidemiology, School of Public Health, University of North Carolina, and a Primary Care Provider who has used his practice as a research base in community medicine. He has received National Institutes of Health funding since 1958. This research project is the longest total, longitudinal, black-white cohort under continuous observation in this country. His main research thrust has been to study simultaneously as many environmental determinants of disease as possible and how they may impact differently on the two cohorts.

**Ronald D. Hays,** Ph.D, is a Scientist at RAND Corporation in Santa Monica, California, and a Senior Statistician at UCLA in the Department of Public Health. He received his bachelor's degree and his doctoral degree from the University of California, Riverside.

**Brian Hennen,** MD, is Chairman of the Department of Family Medicine at The University of Western Ontario. He graduated in medicine from Queen's University in 1962. He was the first recipient of the D. I. Rice Merit Award and one the first 12 certificants of the CFPC in 1969.

**John Howie,** MD, Ph.D., FRCPE, FRCGP, is Professor of General Practice in the University of Edinburgh. While in laboratory medicine he researched into the pathology of abdominal pain and, later as a general practitioner, into antibiotic use in general practice. His present interests are stress in general practice and the relation between the use of time and quality of care. He is author of the book *Research in General Practice*

**Adam Keller,** MPH, is an Instructor in Community and Family Medicine at Dartmouth Medical School, Hanover, New Hampshire, and is Executive Director of the Dartmouth COOP Project. He received his bachelor's degree from Harvard College and his MPH from the University of Minnesota.

**John W. Kirk,** MD, is in private practice of general internal medicine in New London, New Hampshire, and is also President of the medical staff of New London Medical Center. He is board certified in internal and preventive medicine and received his bachelor's degree from Providence College and his MD from Cornell University Medical College.

**Jeanne M. Landgraf,** MA, is a Senior Research Associate at the Institute for the Advancement of Health and Medical Care, New England Medical Center, Boston, Massachusetts. She received her bachelor's and master's degrees from San Diego State University, California.

**Richard A. MacLachlan,** BSc, MD, FCFP, is Medical Director for Camp Hill Medical Centre and Professor in the Department of Family Medicine, Dalhousie University, both in Halifax, Nova Scotia, Canada. Prior to his appointment to Camp Hill Medical Centre in 1990, he was Professor in the Department of Family Medicine at Queen's University, Kingston, Ontario, Canada. He is a member of the National Council on Bioethics in Human Research.

**David Metcalfe,** MB, ChB, FRCGP, FFPHM, is Professor of General Practice at the University of Manchester, England. After 12 years in general practice in England he did 2 years as Assistant Professor of Family Medicine at Rochester, New York, followed by 6 years as Senior Lecturer (GP) in Community Medicine at the New Medical School at Nottingham. His current department at Manchester includes, integrally, a large inner city group practice caring for 13,000 patients, and a Department of Health-funded research unit, the Centre for Primary Care Research, and all three components of the Department have contributed to primary care research with particular emphasis on variations in process of care and patient's perception of health and care.

**William L. Miller,** MD, a Physician-Anthropologist in the Department of Family Medicine at the University of Connecticut, is active in an effort to make qualitative research more accessible to health care researchers. He is coeditor of a quarterly newsletter, *The Interpreter,* funded by the North American Primary Research Group (NAPRG) and has contributed book chapters and articles detailing step-by-step applications of qualitative methods.

**David L. Morgan,** Ph.D., is an Associate Professor in the Institute on Aging at Portland State University. His research interests center on the role that social networks and personal relationships play in coping with role transitions across the life-course. In addition to his book *Focus Groups as Qualitative Research,* his work has appeared in such journals as the *American Journal of Sociology, Journal of Health and Social Behavior, Sociology of Health and Illness,* and *The Gerontologist.*

**Eugene C. Nelson,** ScD, is Director of Quality Care Research at the Hospital Corporation of America and Adjunct Professor at Vanderbilt School of Medicine. With interests in primary care research, quality improvement, health status assessment, outcomes research, and health promotion, he has published in books and such journals as *Journal of the American Medical Association, Medical Care, New England Journal of Medicine, American Journal of Public Health,* and *Quality Review Bulletin.* In addition to work at HCA he serves on research teams based at Dartmouth Medical School (Primary Care Cooperative Research Project) and at New England Medical Center (Medical Outcomes Study). He received his doctoral degree in Health Services from the Harvard School of Public Health.

**Peter G. Norton,** BSc, MA, PhD, MD, CCFP, Associate Professor, Department of Family and Community Medicine, Sunnybrook Health Science Centre, Toronto, Ontario. He came late to family medicine after a first career in mathematics. After his family medicine training he joined the staff of the University of Toronto and helped found the Primary Care Research Unit at Sunnybrook Health Science Centre, a teaching complex owned by the university. His research interests include medical decision making, utilization of health care resources, alternative models of health care delivery, and research methodologies for primary care.

**Truls Østbye,** MD, is a Medical Epidemiologist and Associate Professor in the Department of Epidemiology and Biostatistics at The University of Western Ontario. His research interests include the epidemiology of such diseases as Alzheimer's disease, diabetes, astigmatism, cancer, and hypertension; and health information systems and new teaching methods, particularly by means of computers and electronic communication. His work has been published in such journals as *International Journal of Epidemiology, European Journal of Epidemiology, Journal of the Norwegian Medical Association, Diabetologia,* and *Canadian Family Physician.*

**Moira Stewart,** PhD, Professor in the Centre for Studies in Family Medicine, the Department of Family Medicine at The University of Western Ontario, London, Ontario. With a PhD in Epidemiology, she has conducted research in the primary care setting for the past 15 years, addressing such topics as research methods, quality of care, doctor-patient communication in relation to outcomes, and the association of stress with health. She has published papers in *Social Science and Medicine, The Journal of the Royal College of General Practitioners, Family Practice: An International Journal, the Canadian Medical Association Journal,* and *Medical Care.* She recently edited books titled *Communicating with Medical Patients* and *Primary Care Research-Traditional and Innovative Approaches.*

**Fred Tudiver,** MD, CCFP, is a family physician and Assistant Professor in the Department of Family and Community Medicine at the Sunnybrook Health Science Centre at the University of Toronto, Canada. He has extensive experience in primary prevention—particularily with the use of mutual support and with the creation and use of measures of self-report. He has worked on the evaluation of community-based AIDS health education, support for new widowers, and a new measure for evaluating breast self-examination. His current interests include the content and evaluation of psychotherapy by family physicians; the health care utilization patterns of new widowers; and family physicians' knowledge, attitudes, and practice with respect to wife abuse.

**John H. Wasson,** MD, is Professor of Clinical Community & Family Medicine at Dartmouth Medical School, Hanover, New Hampshire. He is board certified in internal medicine and received his bachelor's degree from Dartmouth College and his MD from the University of Virginia.

**David Wilkin,** Ph.D., is Associate Professor of the Centre for Primary Care Research in the Department of General Practice at the University of Manchester. He is a sociologist with extensive experience of research in the field of health and social care. He has worked on family care of mentally handicapped children, hospital and community services for elderly people, and primary health care. His current interests include the management of chronic illness in general practice, referrals from general practitioners to specialists, community care for elderly and disabled people, and the measurement of outcomes in primary health care. He is the author of a forthcoming book on instruments for the measurement of outcomes in primary health care.

**J. Ivan Williams,** Ph.D., is Deputy Director of the Clinical Epidemiology Unit of the Sunnybrook Health Sciences Centre. He is a Professor at the University of Toronto and holds academic appointments in the Department of Family and Community Medicine, the Department of Preventive Medicine and Biostatistics, and the Faculty of Nursing. His primary research interests are health care evaluation, assessing outcomes, and methods for measuring quality of life. His research projects include quality assessments in family medicine; the evaluation of prehospital emergency services; and related resource use, practice procedures, and outcomes.

**Maurice Wood,** MD, is Professor Emeritus, Department of Family Practice, Virginia Commonwealth University. He has published widely on primary care research issues, including taxonomy. From 1979 he chaired a World Health Organization Working Party to develop a core classification for pri- mary care, which evolved into the *International Classification of Primary Care* (ICPC), published under the aegis of the World Organization of Family Doctors (WONCA).

**Stephen J. Zyzanski,** Ph.D., is Professor of Family Medicine at Case Western Reserve University. His research interests include behavioral medicine and cardiovascular disease epidemiology, primary care and survey research, geriatric and screening studies, and scaling and attitute scale construction. His work has been published in books and journals focusing on primary care and chronic disease research.